The
EVERYTHING®
Pregnancy Fitness Book

Dear Reader:

Congratulations on your upcoming new addition. Whether this is your first baby or your fourth, pregnancy is a time of great change. You might be thinking about how pregnancy will change your body as well as your life. *The Everything® Pregnancy Fitness Book* is designed to help you have a healthy and happy pregnancy, while minimizing the negative effects of a sedentary pregnancy on your body.

Even after you have the baby, this book will help you address body-related issues, such as weight loss and building your strength back up. Not only will you have to learn to deal with a new physical you, but you will also need to learn to find time to keep your body fit and healthy. Within these pages you can find information on making the most of your postpartum workout and exercising with your new baby.

I hope you enjoy the good health and fitness that you will achieve by exercising during this special period in your life. Feel free to drop me a line and show off your baby pictures at ✎ *www.robineliseweiss.com.*

Have a happy and healthy birth!

Robin Elise Weiss

The EVERYTHING® Series

Editorial

Publishing Director	Gary M. Krebs
Managing Editor	Kate McBride
Copy Chief	Laura MacLaughlin
Acquisitions Editor	Eric M. Hall
Development Editor	Patrycja Pasek-Gradziuk
Production Editor	Khrysti Nazzaro
	Jamie Wielgus

Production

Production Director	Susan Beale
Production Manager	Michelle Roy Kelly
Series Designers	Daria Perreault
	Colleen Cunningham
Cover Design	Paul Beatrice
	Frank Rivera
Layout and Graphics	Colleen Cunningham
	Rachael Eiben
	Michelle Roy Kelly
	Daria Perreault
	Erin Ring
Series Cover Designer	Barry Littmann
Cover Illustrations	Marcey Ramsey
Photographer	Brian Moberly

THE
EVERYTHING®
PREGNANCY
FITNESS BOOK

Safe, specially tailored exercises for
before and after delivery

Robin Elise Weiss,
Certified Childbirth Educator

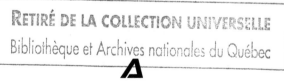

Adams Media
Avon, Massachusetts

To my family: Kevin, Hilary, Benjamin, Isaac, Lilah, Owen, and Clara.

An Everything® Series Book.
Everything® and everything.com® are registered trademarks of F+W Publications, Inc.

Published by Adams Media, an F+W Publications Company
57 Littlefield Street, Avon, MA 02322 U.S.A.
www.adamsmedia.com

ISBN: 1-58062-873-7
Printed in the United States of America.

J I H G F E D C B A

Library of Congress Cataloging-in-Publication Data
Elise Weiss, Robin.
The everything pregnancy fitness book / Robin Elise Weiss.
p.   cm.
(The everything series book)
ISBN 1-58062-873-7
1. Exercise for pregnant women. 2. Physical fitness for women.
I. Title. II. Series: Everything series.
RG558.7.E43 2003
618.2'4—dc21
2003014707

This publication is designed to provide accurate and authoritative information with regard to the subject matter covered. It is sold with the understanding that the publisher is not engaged in rendering legal, accounting, or other professional advice. If legal advice or other expert assistance is required, the services of a competent professional person should be sought.

—From a *Declaration of Principles* jointly adopted by a Committee of the American Bar Association and a Committee of Publishers and Associations

Many of the designations used by manufacturers and sellers to distinguish their products are claimed as trademarks. Where those designations appear in this book and Adams Media was aware of a trademark claim, the designations have been printed with initial capital letters.

The Everything® Pregnancy Fitness Book does not purport to render medical advice. Every pregnant woman should consult her medical professional for such advice.

This book is available at quantity discounts for bulk purchases.
For information, call 1-800-872-5627.

Contents

Acknowledgments

Writing this book has been so much fun! But I have many people to thank for their help and support: Owen and Clara, for testing out the exercises as my babies in utero during the writing of this book; Kim Goldman, Robin Newlon, and Janice Wood, for keeping me well fed and hydrated; Eve Hiatt, for being my editor and friend; Bryan Moberly, for his great photographic works; Whitney and Sarah, for modeling the exercises to bring this book together; and my Mom, for setting the family precedence on authoring books. Thanks also to Barb Doyen, a wonderful agent who showed me the ropes, and Eric Hall, who answered way too many questions for me! Much appreciation goes to Hilary, Benjamin, Isaac, and Lilah for giving up their mom on the weekends so that I could actually write the book. And thanks to Kevin and Amanda for believing I could do it.

Top Ten Things You Will Know
After Reading This Book

1. When you exercise during pregnancy, you will feel better about your newly pregnant shape.

2. Focusing on good health during pregnancy increases your body awareness to prevent preterm labor.

3. If you exercise while pregnant, you will have fewer aches and pains associated with pregnancy.

4. By working out during pregnancy, you are less likely to gain unwanted pounds.

5. Studies show that if you exercise during pregnancy you will tend to have a faster labor.

6. Babies born to women who worked out while pregnant tend to be leaner and calmer than babies born to women who did not exercise.

7. You are less likely to have a cesarean section to give birth if you stay fit during pregnancy.

8. Staying fit during pregnancy leads to a faster weight loss after your baby is born.

9. If you exercise during pregnancy, you can generally resume fitness activities sooner after birth.

10. Working out with your baby makes it more likely that you will stick to an exercise program and stay fit after birth.

Introduction

▶BEING PHYSICALLY FIT is an important part of being a healthy, well-rounded individual. These days, pregnancy and postpartum are the times when more and more families are introduced to regular exercise. It is a time to look out not only for yourself, but for your unborn baby as well.

As science decides that physical fitness and exertion are not only acceptable but also essential parts of a healthy pregnancy, more women are taking part in the physical fitness movement during pregnancy. The result is not only healthier, but also happier moms and babies.

The American College of Obstetricians and Gynecologists (ACOG) highly encourages that women with low-risk pregnancies work out at least three times a week, if not more. Women who are in a high-risk pregnancy or questionable situation can often find a suitable form of exercise with the help of their practitioners.

Exercise has been shown in scientific studies to reduce the amount of weight gained in pregnancy. Furthermore, pregnant women who regularly exercise also report fewer pregnancy-related complaints, such as backaches, sciatica, or muscular cramps. The movements of exercise also help with other pregnancy-induced complications, such as fatigue, a major source of frustration by pregnant women and their families.

Moms who work out also tend to have shorter, easier labors than their counterparts who don't exercise. These labors are also less likely to be plagued by complications or interventions like episiotomies, which are generally done for a couple of reasons. One reason might be if the tissues look likely to tear (as opposed to a practitioner who always cuts one). Tearing is much more common in women who do not have good muscle tone in that area, or good control of those muscles.

Physical exercise in pregnancy has also shown that these exercising moms tend to recover faster from whatever labor brings them—even if it's a cesarean section or an episiotomy.

During the early postpartum period, mothers who worked out during pregnancy are more likely to resume exercise. This means that they also lose their pregnancy weight more easily and at a faster pace. Add breastfeeding, which burns off excess calories and fat deposits, to the exercising, and the weight and fat deposits seem to melt away! Overall, the healthier lifestyle is of benefit to the new family.

Learning to exercise in a safe and effective manner is a key element in any plan. This means that you will need to closely examine your previous exercise and fitness history. By taking this information and discussing your plans and pregnancy with your current doctor or midwife, you can find an appropriate workout plan.

Basically, physical fitness in pregnancy is for everyone, with the proper supervision.

The Everything® Pregnancy Fitness Book will help you find the path that is right for you. From the first trimester to the finish, you've got exercises galore and exercise tips to help keep you motivated and healthy. We've even included ideas to help you continue exercising after the baby comes.

Whether you do aerobics, swim, or walk the dog, exercise is a key element in any healthy pregnancy. Remember to always check with your practitioner before making drastic changes in your workout regimen. Mostly, remember to have fun and find an exercise that keeps you enthused enough to make it a lifelong habit. Ⓔ

Chapter 1

Understanding Pregnancy Fitness

Although fitness during pregnancy is a fairly new concept, the act of keeping healthy during pregnancy has always been a goal. Today's active woman is more likely to include fitness as a part of her healthy prenatal routine than ever before. With the guidelines that have come out as a way to help women maintain their fitness and health during pregnancy, more women are taking advantage of pregnancy fitness.

History of Pregnancy Fitness

It was not long ago that if you were expecting a baby, you were placed on near house arrest. In the delicate condition of "being with child," you would not wish to be seen in public, let alone actually *doing* anything. If you did venture out in public, you did so in garments that were constructed with very tight corsets to hide your expanding abdomen. There was virtually no outlet for physical exertion or exercise.

This confinement was a drastic switch from the pre–Industrial Revolution days when pregnant women continued with their daily lives and activities until their babies were born. Then, after some recuperation time, they went back to their normal duties fairly quickly. Exercise was out of the question. Today, the exercise pendulum has swung the other way as research study after study has shown that fitness is an important part of pregnancy and the prenatal care a woman receives.

Research Opens Eyes

As women came out into society with their pregnant abdomens boldly going where none had gone before, they began to wonder if maintaining fitness during pregnancy was really a lost cause. The research was conducted and women slowly changed their thinking about fitness in pregnancy. More women maintained their previous fitness levels in pregnancy and more research was done. The majority of the research showed that fitness in pregnancy was extremely beneficial in nearly every capacity.

In 1985, the American College of Obstetricians and Gynecologists (ACOG) released their first set of guidelines for pregnancy fitness. These original fitness guidelines were still quite restrictive, although definitely a step in the right direction. Up until this point, not many studies had been done, and the ACOG was erring on the side of caution. As time went by and more studies were completed, the rules for exercise in pregnancy became more lax. Women were able to get out and stay active throughout their pregnancies, and the practitioners were seeing that there was no harm being done to these women, their pregnancies, or their babies.

During the height of the fitness boom of the 1980s, pregnant women wanted to take part, too. With ACOG's guidelines out, they now had something to back them up and so they continued to exercise during pregnancy. The guidelines have since been updated numerous times, each time becoming more lenient. The most recent ACOG guidelines were published in January 2002, suggesting that "an accumulation of 30 minutes or more of moderate exercise a day should occur on most, if not all, days of the week."

According to ACOG, in absence of either medical or obstetric complications, pregnant women can also adopt this recommendation:

"Given the potential risks, albeit rare, thorough clinical evaluation of each pregnant woman should be conducted before recommending an exercise program. In the absence of complications, pregnant women should be encouraged to engage in regular, moderate intensity physical activity to continue to derive the same associated health benefits during their pregnancies as they did prior to their pregnancies."

E ALERT!

When talking to your doctor or midwife about exercise during your pregnancy, be sure to ask if they are familiar with the newest guidelines from the American College of Obstetricians and Gynecologists (ACOG). This can be a useful learning tool for the both of you. A copy can be obtained by writing ACOG at ✍ *resources@acog.org*.

The Green Light

These days, it is not uncommon to see pregnant women exercising everywhere. You will find them in aerobics class. Perhaps you have seen them lifting weights at the gym. They are swimming at the pool. The good news is that pregnancy fitness has obvious health benefits to mom and baby for both short-term and long-term outcomes.

As it stands today, the American College of Obstetricians and Gynecologists (ACOG) recommends that pregnant women exercise for thirty minutes or more, nearly every day of the week, though exercising every day is not a problem. So, get out and get fit!

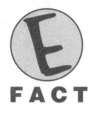

If you exercise during pregnancy, you will tend to have a much faster recovery after childbirth. You will also gain less weight and lose what weight you do gain more quickly than your non-exercising counterparts. Studies also show that you will have a decrease in the length of your labor if you've taken the time to get fit prior to childbirth.

Philosophy of Pregnancy Fitness

While the word *fitness* may bring to mind sweating and buff bodies, this image is not appropriate for pregnancy. Fitness during the nine months of pregnancy is more about health and wellness than at nearly any other point in your life. In fact, many women and their families do not even start on the path to fitness until they become pregnant. This major life change alters the outlook and goals you have in nearly every respect. It is a time to re-evaluate your priorities for a healthy lifestyle.

The goals of pregnancy fitness are to maintain the strength and wellness that you currently have, while preventing physical problems from occurring. For the woman who is already very fit this might mean actually slowing down a normal workout as the pregnancy advances. Clearly, if you are just starting a fitness program, exercise will be an increase in your activity. Though an increase in activity should not be a drastic one, as pregnancy is not the time to rebuild your body, you can still safely begin a fitness program during pregnancy. As you look at the benefits of exercising while pregnant, it is very obvious what the answer should be: Just do it!

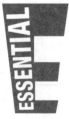

If you are used to exercise, continuing down that path in pregnancy is natural. For those who have not exercised before it may be more difficult. Amanda Ralston, one mother, remembers that getting out and walking was the best thing she could do. It kept her from sitting on the couch but did not require a lot of planning or effort. It also led to a continuing passion for walking after the birth of her baby.

The Physiological Effects

There is a lot of medical literature available on exercise in general. While everyone knows that exercise is good for you, it does not mean we all participate in it. Now that it has been established that exercise is good, even for an expectant woman, we are finding that more and more women are getting out and getting fit, or staying fit during pregnancy.

The physiological benefits of exercise on pregnancy are great. Not only can exercise change the course of your pregnancy and of your labor, but it can also help you reduce stress. The benefits also go well into the postpartum period and beyond.

Body awareness is a key component to exercise in pregnancy (and pregnancy in general!). As you begin to exercise, your body awareness increases. This attention to your body can help you become more attuned to problems before they become larger issues. This can in turn lead to an increase in attention to proper body mechanics and body posture, both of which are key to a comfortable pregnancy.

Physical Complaints

The physical complaints of pregnancy are many. Among the most often-heard complaints are fatigue, backache, digestion problems, constipation, and swelling. Exercise can help you prevent many of these complaints for a variety of reasons.

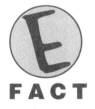

FACT

Backache in pregnancy is one of the most common complaints women have. Not only does exercise help with alleviating back pain, but it also helps prevent back pain from occurring to begin with, and makes caring for your baby easier after the birth because your muscles are more used to being held appropriately.

Reducing Fatigue and Strength Building

The physical movements of exercise can help you combat the fatigue that is so common in the first and third trimesters. Additionally, exercise helps alleviate problems with insomnia that can also plague pregnant women at all stages of pregnancy and recovery.

When you physically utilize your body during the day, your body responds by requiring a recuperation period. The physical demands of exercise, even when not intense, will also help you clear your mind and rest more easily at night.

Certain exercises also increase the strength and the flexibility of your body, which will be very handy advantages for the physical demands of pregnancy and labor. This added strength and mobility will also make the tasks of caring for a newborn seem less extreme. All of these events use muscles you never knew you had!

Blood Volume Increase

When you are pregnant, you experience an increase in your blood volume, as much as 50 percent of your blood volume with one baby and more if you are carrying multiples. Exercise also helps increase the circulation of your blood, which can prevent a number of circulatory issues common to pregnancy: varicose veins of the legs and rectum (hemorrhoids), blood clots that occur during pregnancy and after, and some forms of swelling associated with pregnancy.

Physical Benefits of Exercise

The improved body awareness that you gain from exercising will help you manage the physical symptoms of pregnancy with greater ease. This directly corresponds with feeling more comfortable as your body goes through the many changes of the three trimesters. Exercising will also decrease the number of physical complaints commonly associated with pregnancy.

Other physical benefits of exercise in pregnancy include:

- Decrease in headaches
- Decrease in shortness of breath
- Improved digestion
- Improved bowel function
- Increased sense of well-being
- Decreased tendency toward depression

- Maintained or improved cardiovascular strength
- Increased pelvic floor strength
- Improved posture
- Better sense of control over body issues

Weight Gain in Pregnancy

You might be dreading the thought of putting on weight during pregnancy despite the fact that the weight you will gain will not be all fat, nor will it be a bad thing. The dramatic weight gain of pregnancy is just something that bothers many women. How you deal with the normal and expected weight gain will depend on your understanding of the physiology of a normal, healthy pregnancy. Knowing that pregnancy weight gain is not only normal, but also expected, can help you address issues that you must face going forward in your pregnancy.

How Much Weight and Where Does It Go?

Gone are the days when women were restricted to 10 or 15 pounds of weight gain during pregnancy. Instead your doctor or midwife will likely expect you to gain between 25 and 45 pounds during the course of your pregnancy. If you are expecting twins, you will be expected to gain between 45 and 65 pounds during your pregnancy. There might be reasons for you to gain more or less, but this should only be done with the supervision of your practitioner.

This positive approach to weight gain in pregnancy is not only beneficial for you, but your baby as well. Inadequate weight gain in pregnancy has been associated with preterm birth, poor placental function, and other negative outcomes. To give your baby the best start possible, you need to gain weight—wisely. Keeping in mind that your baby needs every bite of food you take in will help you as you adjust your dietary intake.

Gaining weight during pregnancy is usually not a hard task. If you experience problems with nausea or vomiting in the beginning of your pregnancy, you might take longer to show a weight gain. In fact, you might even show up to a prenatal appointment and be surprised to see that the scale has moved down! This can be fairly normal. As long as you and baby are both growing, the actual numbers from week to week are not of concern.

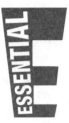

Calorie counting is important in pregnancy, although the number of actual calories you need is probably not as high as you would think. In the average pregnancy with one baby you will need to add about 300 calories a day to your diet, which is basically one extra snack. Examples might be a half of a peanut butter sandwich, or cheese and crackers.

Our society tends to think of pregnancy weight gain going directly to your belly. A typical pregnant woman has a large abdomen and a regular body. Therefore, you might not realize where the weight gain in pregnancy is distributed throughout your body. A typical weight distribution for a pregnant woman might look like this:

7½ to 8½ pounds	Baby
2 pounds	Amniotic fluid
2 pounds	Placenta
1½ to 2 pounds	Breast tissue
3 pounds	Blood volume
2 to 2½ pounds	Uterine tissues
4 pounds	Water
8 pounds	Fat stores
30–32 pounds	**TOTAL**

Weight Gain Distribution

Now that you know exercise in pregnancy can counterbalance the amount of unnecessary weight gain, along with proper nutrition habits it will also help you to avoid excessive or unnecessary accumulation of fatty deposits often associated with pregnancy. Weight gain is usually distributed unevenly during pregnancy. This is not a cause for worry. Here is an average way to look at weight gain distribution in pregnancy:

- Between 2 and 5 pounds in the first twenty weeks for a singleton pregnancy
- ½ to 1 pound per week until birth for a singleton pregnancy

If you were underweight before becoming pregnant, a larger weight gain may be appropriate for you and is generally recommended. For instance, if you were expected to normally gain between 25 and 35 pounds during pregnancy, you can probably expect to add 5 to 10 pounds to that total to make up for starting your pregnancy at a lower weight. Your doctor or midwife can help you determine a proper weight gain for your body. This additional weight will help ensure a healthy pregnancy.

If you are overweight, it is never expected that you will gain less than 20 pounds during pregnancy. Lowered weight gains in overweight women have been shown to produce smaller, sicklier babies who are often born premature. These outcomes are best avoided by adequate intake of calories. Even if you are obese, you must gain weight in pregnancy. Dieting in pregnancy is never appropriate.

Eating Disorders and Weight Gain

If you have previously suffered from an eating disorder such as anorexia nervosa or bulimia, you need to share this information with your doctor or midwife. Having a history of an eating disorder does put you in a higher risk category for problems with weight gain during pregnancy. Your practitioner can help you deal with issues concerning weight gain before they become an issue. Counseling might also be recommended. The good news is that even if you've previously suffered from an eating disorder, you can still have a healthy pregnancy.

Labor and Birth Advantages

While we tend to want immediate gratification from everything we do, exercise in pregnancy doesn't always fall into this category. Sometimes it can be difficult to get up and exercise when the benefits aren't seen immediately. However, the exercises you do in pregnancy will certainly affect how you give birth when the time comes.

Having a well-toned and fit body for labor has its advantages. If you have been used to the physical rigors of exercise, you will tend to do better in labor. You will be more prepared for the physical demands placed on your body. The strength that you will need for pushing and the muscles that have been prepared, perhaps even specifically for the task of labor and birth, are more easily put into action.

Beyond the feelings of having more strength and stamina, there are some specific benefits to you for exercising in pregnancy. Studies have shown that women who exercise during pregnancy often have shorter labors. These women also tend to require cesarean surgery less often, as well as experiencing a decrease in the use of forceps and vacuum extractors. By decreasing the risks of surgery and instrumental deliveries, you will also speed your recovery period.

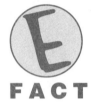

FACT

Some childbirth classes will offer a few exercises to incorporate into your exercise habits. These exercises are usually specially designed to prepare specific muscles in your body for labor and birth. An example might be teaching the class about squatting. It's a great exercise to strengthen your legs and "glutes" (buttocks), but is also the perfect position to actually give birth in as it opens the pelvic outlet by an additional 10 percent.

Postpartum Advantages

Possibly some of the most surprising benefits of exercise in pregnancy are the postpartum benefits. If you've spent time building strength and flexibility during pregnancy, you will tend to have an easier recovery period after the birth of your baby. Coupled with the fact that you will tend to have an easier birth with fewer cesareans and episiotomies, it makes sense.

Not only is exercise beneficial in terms of your weight loss, but in your body tone and fitness levels in general. Returning to your pre-pregnancy body is a huge issue for women in the postpartum period. When you stay fit before birth, you have a huge leap ahead of the crowd toward getting your old body back. There also seems to be a protective benefit from postpartum depression when you have exercised during pregnancy.

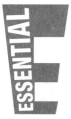

You might be concerned with losing weight after the birth of your baby. Did you know that one of the best ways to lose weight after baby is to breastfeed your infant? The fat stores your body has accumulated during pregnancy are designed to be used for breastfeeding.

The Psychological Effects

By now, you have read a lot of information about the physical benefits of exercise for you and your baby in different periods during the childbearing year. But there are many emotional and mental benefits as well to gain from exercise. It has long been shown that, in general, exercising helps to lower your stress levels. This stress reduction is very important during such a tense, albeit happy, time in your life.

There is an increased pride in your pregnancy and your pregnant body when you are physically meeting your body's needs through exercise. This sense of confidence and self-esteem that comes from exercise helps you envision your newly rounding figure with pride and pleasure. No longer do you see yourself as a "beached whale" awaiting the delivery of your calf. You now see the beauty and function of your new pregnant form. This is just another benefit of knowing the body you live in.

Finally, as exercise becomes a part of your way of life, it becomes a habit, a healthy habit that can be shared as a family. Exercising moms rarely just quit exercising after the birth of their babies. They begin exercising *with* their babies. This starts the baby on a lifelong journey to seek out fitness for himself or herself, because it is what he or she has learned by Mom's great example.

The Effects on Baby

In the past, one of the main concerns about exercise during pregnancy was that it would have a negative effect on your baby. Some researchers predicted growth restriction, oxygen reduction, and other scary outcomes for babies born to moms who exercised. To the contrary, researchers have now found that there are many physical and psychological benefits for a baby when Mom exercises during pregnancy.

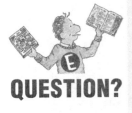

QUESTION?

How can I monitor my baby's well-being?
Your practitioner will monitor your baby in a couple of ways during your pregnancy. One way will be by measuring the heart rate; another is the growth rate as judged by the growth of your uterus. Your baby's normal heart rate will probably be between 120 and 160 beats per minute (bpm). After twenty weeks, your uterus will generally measure within one to two weeks of the number of weeks you are pregnant. The measurements are in centimeters, from the public bone to the top of the fundus.

As you become more aware of your pregnant body and your baby, you focus on taking proper care of that body and baby. By watching how and what you eat, you decrease the risks of preterm labor. The decrease in preterm birth rates alone prevents many neonatal deaths, as preterm birth is one of the leading causes of death in newborns.

Healthier Placenta

The improved blood circulation of the mother through exercise can help grow a healthier placenta, which is the baby's lifeline during pregnancy, as it uses the placenta to get nutrients and oxygen and to expel waste products. The heartier the placenta, the healthier the baby will be.

Improved Labor Tolerance

Babies of mothers who exercise also seem to tolerate labor better. These babies are used to having Mom work hard while exercising, so that when it is time for Mom to have contractions—it is just another workout for them. This tolerance level has also shown to decrease the incidence of meconium (baby's first stool) in the amniotic fluid at birth. Having too much meconium in the amniotic fluid is potentially life-threatening and something you would prefer to avoid.

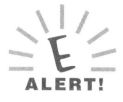

ALERT!

You can also monitor your baby between prenatal visits using fetal kick counts. At the same time every day, relax for thirty minutes and notice how long it takes Baby to reach ten movements. It should take about the same amount of time each day, usually less than an hour. If an hour is up and you need more movements, eat something and try again. If there is still a decrease or change in the number of movements, report it immediately to your doctor or midwife.

Leaner, Healthier Babies

If you exercise during pregnancy, your baby will tend to be of a lower birth weight. While this might seem like a negative outcome, the lower weight is not from fetal growth restriction, but rather the reduction in deposits of unnecessary fat for the baby. These leaner babies at birth are also healthier and leaner later in life. Some studies even report that babies born to mothers who exercised during pregnancy were easier to care for after birth and seemed to adjust to their environments more readily.

Perhaps these babies are reported to be easier because the rocking motions associated with maternal exercise during pregnancy offered stimulation to enhance baby's brain development. One study, "Morphometric and neurodevelopmental outcome at age five years of the offspring of women who continued to exercise regularly throughout pregnancy" (*J. Pediatr.* 1996 Dec; 129[6]:856-63), shows that these babies actually had better language and intelligence scores at five years of life.

It is clear, then, that babies enjoy many benefits from having a healthy mother and a healthy pregnancy. They are heartier and healthier. They also seem to do better than other babies in a similar situation.

Recent studies have shown that exercise in pregnancy is a safe and effective way to maintain a healthy pregnancy. While this has not always been the thinking, we now see the benefits to maintaining the strength and flexibility of the pregnant body. You and your baby have many benefits to gain.

Chapter 2

When Is Exercise Appropriate in Pregnancy?

Given the benefits of exercise to you, your pregnancy, and your baby, it is clear that prenatal exercise is a good thing. However, it is important to approach exercise in pregnancy with a level head. Just as you should know when to exercise, it is also wise to know what to avoid when exercising. The key is to strike a balance—to reap the benefits of exercise in pregnancy without compromising your health or the health of your baby.

Knowing When Not to Exercise

It seems that there is always a reason not to exercise. We are all busy with our families and work. This is not to mention our other commitments to outside sources, so common to everyday life. However, exercise should be a priority in your life and not an afterthought.

That said, there are some valid reasons exercise may not be appropriate for you during pregnancy. Sometimes you will be asked to avoid exercise, or certain exercises during certain periods of pregnancy, while other problems may preclude you from exercising your entire pregnancy. The decision of what exercise is appropriate for you and when you should start your exercise program is best discussed with your doctor or midwife during your regular prenatal visits.

ESSENTIAL

If you suffer from certain chronic conditions such as thyroid issues, heart problems, hypertension, or diabetes, you will want to discuss your fitness needs with your medical team. These conditions are not necessarily absolute reasons not to exercise, but they will require careful monitoring.

Warning Signs

While there are not many reasons that exercise would be contraindicated during pregnancy, it is important to know what to look for in terms of protecting yourself. In general, here are some problems that you may experience that would signal you to stop exercise during portions or all of your pregnancy.

Bleeding

About 30 to 40 percent of women will experience some form of bleeding during pregnancy. The majority of these women, more than 60 percent, will go on to carry a healthy baby to the end of pregnancy. However, it is wise to find out the source of the bleeding, which will determine whether or not you can exercise.

For example, the cervix region becomes much more vascular during pregnancy. Sometimes something as simple as a vaginal exam or sexual intercourse can cause the cervix to bleed slightly. While this is definitely scary, it does not necessarily mean an impending miscarriage or other problems with the pregnancy. However, bleeding from the uterus, like under the placenta, also called a *partial abruption*, would be a reason not to exercise during this pregnancy until the issues were resolved and your doctor or midwife gave you the go-ahead.

Placenta previa is a condition in which part of or the entire placenta covers the opening of the uterus, the cervix. This can lead to bleeding, with or without pain, as well as pregnancy loss and other trauma to the pregnancy. There may not be an opportunity for you to exercise during this type of pregnancy because of the inherent risks. Ask your provider about how this will affect your pregnancy and birth. You might also ask how often and how they intend to monitor the location of the placenta. Many times this condition will spontaneously resolve itself during the second trimester as the body of the uterus grows, helping to move the placenta away from the cervix.

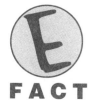

FACT

Placenta previa, detected via ultrasound prior to twenty weeks of gestation, often does not wind up interfering with the birth process. As you enter the second trimester, the body of the uterus begins a major growth spurt, often helping the placenta to move from the cervical region in 95 percent of the women. If the placenta does not move far enough away, your baby will be born via a cesarean surgery.

History of Preterm Labor

If you have previously given birth to a baby before thirty-seven weeks, you will want to talk to your practitioner about exercise. In certain cases, your previous birth may have had a non-repeating factor that caused you to have your baby early. This means that this particular pregnancy is not at a higher risk for preterm birth. Some practitioners, however, will advise that exercise for the first portion of pregnancy is best avoided to confirm the fact that it was a non-repeating factor. And then again, they may advise taking it easy during the later portion of pregnancy.

Contractions

The rhythmic tightening of the uterus that leads to cervical changes is not good; if you feel it, you should discontinue exercising immediately. These contractions are an indicator of preterm labor, even if they are not painful or even noticeable. Any regularly occurring contractions you feel prior to thirty-seven weeks of pregnancy should be immediately reported to your doctor or midwife.

Incompetent Cervix

Incompetent cervix is a condition in which your cervix dilates prior to being full term. This can happen with or without noticeable contractions. You may have been previously diagnosed an incompetent cervix in this or a previous pregnancy, in which case you will probably be treated with a cervical cerclage, a stitch placed in the cervix to attempt to delay labor. Exercise is usually contraindicated because of the risk of preterm labor.

Membrane Ruptures

If your water breaks you will likely be confined to bed rest for the remainder of your pregnancy in an attempt to prevent the preterm birth of your baby. While on bed rest, there may be opportunities to do certain types of physical therapy to help prevent muscle loss. Talk to your medical team about utilizing these services. Regular exercise is simply not possible.

It can be perfectly normal to have slight contractions for about twenty to thirty minutes after exercising. However, the contractions that do not stop after this short period of time or those that become very painful or intense need to be reported to your practitioner. Drinking water and lying on your left side should also help contractions decrease in frequency.

Pregnancy Induced Hypertension (PIH)

When your blood pressure is elevated in pregnancy, one must worry about the effects on mom and baby. Overall, exercise will tend to lower blood pressure, but during the actual exercise it does raise your blood pressure. Some practitioners advise that you avoid all exercise if you experience any episode of high blood pressure. Other practitioners take a wait-and-see approach, often depending on the severity of your symptoms and the timing of the onset of the symptoms.

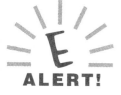
ALERT!

Timing contractions is very simple. Using a watch with a second hand, make a note of when a contraction begins. When the contraction ends, make note of that time as well. The third number to write down will be when the next contraction starts. The period from the beginning of the first contraction to the beginning of the second contraction is how far apart your contractions are. How long they last is from the beginning of one contraction until it ends.

Multiple Gestation

When you are carrying more than one baby, it is simply not well studied as to whether or not exercise is acceptable or beneficial. The general consensus is that with twins, moderate exercise in the beginning of pregnancy is acceptable. Since you will be more closely monitored during the second half of pregnancy, you can look for signs of impending preterm birth, like a shortening cervix. This will alert you and your provider to what changes you need to make in your physical activity levels.

In the later portion of pregnancy, exercise will have to be considered on a case-by-case basis. For those women carrying more than two babies, higher order multiples (HOM), greater restrictions on exercise during pregnancy will exist. However, physical therapy and some forms of stretching may be perfectly acceptable. Again, working with your practitioner is the best option.

Some of these conditions might not make exercise impossible for you, though you may wish to consider modifying your program. It's very important to discuss your current fitness status with your doctor or midwife.

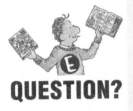

QUESTION?

Are there exercises I should avoid during pregnancy?
Absolutely! A few sports are considered inappropriate during any phase of pregnancy. Mostly these sports are dangerous for reasons related to balance and risk of physical blows. It is not recommended that pregnant women ride horses, scuba dive, downhill ski, play rugby, or engage in other contact sports.

How to Know When to Stop

We have all heard the "no pain, no gain" mantra that is so common in health centers today. And as a society, we all seem too eager to buy into that theory. While it is true that you have to expend energy to get the benefit of exercise, pain has no place in exercise, particularly during pregnancy.

Pain

Pain is your body's way of saying something is wrong. When you are pregnant, it is even more important that you pay attention to these signals from your body. Remember, your baby is counting on you to listen.

Pain should be something that makes you stop exercising immediately. No matter where the location of the pain or what the feeling is like, stop doing whatever you are doing. Sometimes pain is a signal that you have a hurt muscle or a leg cramp. While these may not have a direct negative effect on your pregnancy, they can harm your body.

This type of cramping pain may be more likely to occur during pregnancy. For example, if you have a leg cramp, it may be a sign that your electrolytes are out of balance and that you need to watch your nutritional intake more closely or stretch more often. An injured muscle could result from your body's release of the hormone relaxin, which helps to facilitate the birth but also has the effect of making injuries more likely.

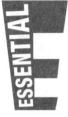

Hormones released during pregnancy, like relaxin, make it more likely for you to pull or strain muscles. By avoiding jerking and bouncing motions during exercise, you can help protect yourself from unnecessary pain and injury.

Falls

Due to the changes in your center of gravity and the hormones coursing through your body, falls may be more likely when pregnant. For this reason, some exercises (e.g., horseback riding) are never recommended during pregnancy.

While you may be at an increased risk for falls, learning to take certain precautions can certainly help reduce this likelihood. During your normal daily life avoid high heels, walk on pathways whenever you can, and avoid uneven surfaces or stones. Whenever you work out, remember to wear the appropriate footwear.

If you do fall, try not to panic. Check yourself out completely before standing back up. In general, your baby is well protected by the amniotic sac in your uterus. However, if you experience any abdominal pain, bleeding, contractions, or changes in the baby's movements, report this immediately to your practitioner.

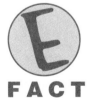

You've just tumbled down the steps for the third time this week. Every time you turn a corner, you forget your belly is larger than it used to be and you bump into walls with it. You are not alone— every pregnant woman feels like a klutz. How can you not? Fear not, though. You will return to your graceful self once your baby is born.

Feeling Weak or Dizzy

Feeling weak or dizzy is a sign that you probably need to skip your exercise today. These feelings can be a normal part of your pregnancy, or they may indicate a problem. Sometimes you feel weak from the exhaustion of pregnancy, more typically in the first and third trimesters. Other issues for feeling weak or dizzy would be a dramatic fluctuation in your blood sugar levels.

If you begin to feel weak or lightheaded during your workout, stop immediately. Sit down or lie down. Have someone bring you water. You should not try to drive or walk. If you actually pass out, be sure to call your doctor or midwife as soon as you awake. Call your doctor or midwife right away if the symptoms don't go away within a few minutes. Otherwise, report your symptoms to your practitioner during normal office hours. They may suggest you alter your exercise plan going forward.

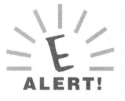

ALERT!

Remember to eat a little something a few hours before you work out. But don't pig out! This can also make you feel ill. Some yogurt and a piece of fruit is just the right thing. This will help your body have the energy you need to sustain your energy through your fitness session.

Sometimes simply not feeling right is a perfect indicator to stop. It could be you're having an off day. Maybe you've not eaten recently enough or perhaps you're tired. Whatever the reason, listen to your body and stop exercising.

The Talk Test

The "talk test" is one of the simpler ways for you to determine whether or not you are exercising at the right intensity for your body and your baby. It is much easier to do than taking your pulse and can be done without any equipment and at any location.

The only thing you have to do is to ask yourself whether you can carry on a conversation with the person next to you without sounding out of breath or winded? It's as simple as that.

So, if, for example, you are out walking with your family or friends in your neighborhood and you are discussing weekend plans, can you do this without huffing and puffing? Or do you sound like you are in need of a breathing machine? If you can carry on the conversation without being winded, you are exercising at the appropriate intensity for you.

ESSENTIAL

While exercising, it is normal to be somewhat out of breath. You should exert yourself enough to work your heart and lungs out during your exercise sessions. The difference between a good windedness and being too short of breath is going to be your ability to carry on a conversation, either real or imagined. Talk to yourself if you need to, just to check yourself.

Now, what do you do if you are winded? Very simple—slow it down. This doesn't mean coming to a complete stop (unless it's severe), but rather shorten your strides when walking and drop the pace, even if this means you fall behind the group. If you are doing aerobics, you might consider doing only leg motions and keeping your arms at your sides instead of including them in the workout, too. If that doesn't work, you can also try walking in place until you can talk at a normal conversational pattern.

When conversation has returned to a normal pace, slowly add speed or activity to what you are doing, being careful not to overexert yourself again. Remember, as you exercise more, your tolerance will increase. The walking pace that winded you last week might this week be perfect.

Risk Factors

There are certain risk factors that predispose you to potential complications while exercising during pregnancy. These potential happenings are usually not a problem if you take the proper precautions. The key in preparing for and preventing mishaps is to look ahead, to know changes you can expect in your pregnant body.

Center of Gravity

Your center of gravity is located in the middle of your abdomen, just above your belly button or umbilicus. Usually, you will not notice any changes to this area until you are into your third or fourth month of pregnancy. Once your uterus has begun to grow out of your pelvic region, your center of gravity will shift upward.

This shift itself is not painful, nor is it cause for alarm. In fact, you will probably not even notice the changes taking place, as it is a gradual process. Your body will naturally adapt to most center of gravity changes. What you do need to watch for is the natural loss of balance that may occur that will probably continue throughout pregnancy, steadily growing as your abdomen does.

ALERT!

It's always wise to wear the appropriate footwear. This goes for times of exercise as well as in everyday life. A simple fall can shake you and leave you feeling unsteady. Don't let your footwear be the cause of it. In addition, always be aware of your surroundings. Watch out for loose flooring, slip rugs, and other objects that are easy to trip on.

Many women report that they feel off balance as their abdomen grows. You might experience this as well. The biggest danger is that the shift makes falls more likely. The good news is that even a serious fall is generally not harmful to your baby. He or she is tucked safely away in the amniotic sac, blissfully unaware of your most recent belly flop. A shift in the center of gravity is more likely to cause problems with your posture as well. Posture is key to feeling good and looking good during your pregnancy. While exercising, simply be aware of your abdomen and try to remain conscious of the movements you are making and how you are moving. This awareness can help with any problems you might experience.

Joints and Flexibility

As with everything in pregnancy, your joints are also affected. This includes your elbows, shoulders, hips, knees, wrists, and ankles. The usual culprits, your hormones, namely relaxin, are to blame for the increased risk of injury to these areas.

Joints can be injured very easily during pregnancy. Using the warmup sessions and cool-downs, you can greatly reduce the risk of harming the joints during pregnancy. These exercises also have the added benefits of working your range of motion.

Previous Exercise Status

You can't pay attention to previous exercise habits enough during pregnancy. While it's perfectly acceptable to begin a mild exercise program if you've never exercised before, the problem is more with people who are used to exercising frequently prior to pregnancy. For these people, there is often a fear of exercising to the point of a good workout. If you've been exercising before your pregnancy, you can probably do the same workouts with only a few modifications for added safety. This is something that can be decided by taking cues from your body, your baby, and your practitioner.

Talking to Your Practitioner about Exercise

Talking with your doctor or midwife about exercise might seem way down on your list of things to discuss in the precious few minutes you have during a regular prenatal appointment. But you can't afford *not* to talk about this issue. Looking at the benefits of pregnancy exercise, you now know it is important to exercise, but it is also crucial that you receive guidance from those taking care of you during your pregnancy.

Ask your practitioner his or her opinion on exercise during pregnancy. Does she seem to agree with the current guidelines for pregnancy fitness released by the American College of Obstetricians and Gynecologists (ACOG)? If she doesn't, ask if there is a specific reason you should not exercise or should not exercise to the extent that you believe you should be able to during this pregnancy.

If she doesn't seem to have an answer that is satisfactory, ask her if she is aware of the latest guidelines from ACOG. If she is not aware, offer to share your copy. This education process can benefit not only you, but also other patients who are seeing this practitioner.

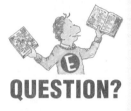

QUESTION?

What if my practitioner refuses to follow the new guidelines?
If you and your practitioner can't see eye to eye about exercise, you may have bigger troubles looming. Remember that you are the consumer and that you can switch practitioners to someone who is supportive of your decisions concerning exercise. If you can't decide together on this issue, you may not be able to agree on other important decisions later, such as medication during labor, genetic testing, and so on.

Maybe you're one of the lucky women who has a practitioner who is very up-to-date on the latest exercise guidelines and is actually encouraging you. Perhaps your provider has a belief in exercise that exceeds the ACOG guidelines. Finding a happy medium—the middle of the road that both you and your practitioner can live with—goes both ways. Talking to your doctor or midwife will help you tailor a fitness program for you and your baby that is safe and effective. This will help ensure a healthy and safe pregnancy fitness course. Ⓔ

Chapter 3

Getting Ready to Exercise

Exercise during pregnancy certainly looks simple. It should be simple; it does not have to be complicated to be effective. Staying fit in pregnancy requires a little preparation on your part, mainly in the form of gathering some good information and developing a team approach with your care provider. As previously stated, this helps you ensure a safe and productive workout throughout your entire pregnancy. Good preparation and planning is what keeps exercise in the prenatal period safe.

Defining Fitness Levels

A fitness level is simply defined as what "shape" your body is in, meaning how fit you are on a cardiovascular level as well as your level of muscle tone. To gauge your fitness level, you might look at how often you exercise. Do you walk every day? Perhaps you take one aerobics class per week. Maybe you get in six exercise sessions a week and if you don't, you feel awful. Each of these categories would represent a different fitness level.

The importance of a fitness evaluation cannot be understated. Choosing a place to start your activity will depend largely on this evaluation. How successful and safe your performance is will also be attributed to the proper determination of your pre-pregnancy fitness level.

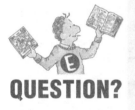

QUESTION?

What if I've never worked out before?
Don't worry! There will be something for you to do as well. Many women start thinking about exercise as they start their families. You just need to be extra alert and careful about the exercises you choose and watch your body's reactions to those choices.

What Is Your Fitness Level?

Finding your fitness level is the first step in any pregnancy or pre-pregnancy exercise program. By using some simple questions about your fitness level, you can then decide on the appropriate place to begin for your current pregnancy. An evaluation should be done with each pregnancy, as your fitness level will change throughout your life.

One of the most important elements of the evaluation, however, will not be which category you are in, but rather your determination and dedication to the exercise program. Remember that intermittent exercise can be more harmful to your body than no exercise at all.

When you exercise irregularly, you're always in the initial phases of exercise. You never really build up to anything, as you can't get past the initial stages of the training. There are also mental reasons why irregular exercise is harmful—because it never gets "any better." You are always doing something that feels difficult to do. This can make you lack the desire to exercise and can also make you more prone to injury.

Let's look at three main fitness levels that will help you define where you fit in: sedentary, moderately active, and athletic.

Sedentary

If you are sedentary, you probably have not been participating in any type of formal exercise program. You may not exercise at all, or very little. Just because you fit into these criteria does not mean that you are necessarily overweight or unhealthy. You might simply just not be as fit as you potentially could be.

Moderately Active

Do you consider yourself moderately active? If so, you probably enjoy exercise but do not go out of your way to make it a regular part of your life. You may exercise when it is convenient or fits into your social schedule, like a walk in the neighborhood with a friend, or a random aerobics or yoga class. You are more likely to add small portions of exercise to your life, like walking short distances rather than driving or parking in the back of the parking lot. This category is more for the social exerciser.

Athletic

You would know if you were classified as an athlete, although this category is not restricted to only professional athletes. You value your exercise highly and would be very lost without your regular routine. Perhaps you go to a regular exercise class or schedule exercise on a near daily basis. You may be a competitive athlete, or perhaps you may compete in more than one sport.

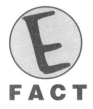

It used to be said that athletes should quit competing when a pregnancy was confirmed. Now we see many pregnant athletes enjoying their sports well into their pregnancy. If you have been athletic prior to pregnancy, barring health issues with the pregnancy, there are few reasons you would need to change your athletic ways.

Assessing Your Needs and Abilities

Looking at these three categories of fitness, you might think you fit neatly into one of them. However, you should only use the fitness level category as a starting point.

Professional Evaluation

Some women prefer to have a professional evaluation of their fitness level. This can be done in most major fitness centers, including some hospital gyms. If you are having trouble finding someone to perform this assessment, you might try a professional association that trains fitness instructors or personal trainers. Fitness evaluation is a basic skill of personal trainers and fitness instructors.

E ALERT!

If you choose to have a professional evaluation, be sure to ask your evaluator about his or her certification in this area. Choosing a certified fitness instructor or personal trainer might make a huge difference in your evaluation.

A few practitioners might require a professional evaluation before giving you the go-ahead to exercise. If your doctor or midwife requests one from you, ask if he or she has a recommendation for where to have your fitness levels tested. In most cases, you will be able to use self-evaluation to figure out where to begin your exercise routine.

Self-Evaluation

Begin your self-evaluation by asking yourself the following questions about your body, your pregnancy, and exercise:

- What injuries have you experienced in the past (including broken bones, accidents, falls, previous surgeries, or other problems)?
- Do you have old injuries that still require nurturing? If so, can you find ways to alter different exercises to accommodate this injury?
- What medical conditions, if any, did you have before your pregnancy

(e.g., chronic conditions including high blood pressure, heart disease, diabetes, arthritis, etc.)? Are they under control now? Do you have any specific concerns about these conditions?

- Are you suffering from current pregnancy discomforts (e.g., swelling, nausea, backache, etc.)?
- Have you developed potential complications during pregnancy, like gestational diabetes, anemia, or pregnancy induced hypertension (PIH)? If so, how can you still fit in exercise? Will there be restrictions on which exercises you are able to complete?

Regular Consultation with Your Practitioner

You will be meeting with your practitioner often throughout pregnancy. Initially, your visits will be monthly, and then later they will become weekly, so there will be an opportunity for constant re-evaluation during pregnancy. Your practitioner can help guide you as you grow in your pregnant body and continue to exercise.

ESSENTIAL

Have you had trouble sticking to an exercise program before? The best advice is to find an exercise buddy to help you stay motivated to exercise. This person doesn't have to be pregnant, but he or she has to be someone on whom you can call for support. It does help if he or she can exercise with you, though this is not a must. The important part of this relationship will be accountability.

Your practitioner will be able to answer questions about the need for changes in your exercise plans and about how to help you accommodate your growing body. Never hesitate to talk to him or her about your questions and concerns.

Finding Time to Exercise

Now down to the nitty-gritty. You know that exercising will be good for you, but where will you find the time? Not having time to exercise is reported as one of the most common reasons for people to quit exercising. Don't let it be your hurdle.

What you need to ask yourself is whether you have the time *not* to exercise? When you are dragging around trying to find excuses not to exercise, remember all those health benefits to you and your baby and the negative outcomes of not exercising.

Making a Schedule

One of the best secrets to finding the time to exercise is to schedule the time. Many women find that if they select a morning time, the exercise gets done. If you wait to do your exercise after work or before bed, things might come up during the day making it easily forgotten. Write the time in your planning calendar—and be faithful to it!

ESSENTIAL

Picking a gym can be a big decision. You should shop around for a gym that you can stay at for a while. For example, don't pick a gym based solely on the prenatal classes. What about a nursery? Can you bring the baby back with you once he or she is born? Look at location in relation to your home or work. What would keep you from coming to the gym? What would make you go?

What if you don't quite feel up to it one day? Or what if you have trouble getting out of bed? Simply get up and do a modified program. Perhaps instead of doing an aerobics tape, you choose to walk the dog leisurely around the block. You are still committing yourself to exercise.

Scheduling the time to exercise into your day is the best way to ensure that you stick to your plan. Just as you make the time to nourish your body with food, be sure to find time to nourish your body with exercise.

Adding Exercise to Your Daily Life

Perhaps there are times when you simply cannot fit exercise into a hectic life, despite scheduling. As long as this does not become a habit, never fear! Find sneaky ways to add exercise into your schedule on the fly. You will be surprised at how easy it can be.

Creative Workouts

Skip the elevator! You should consider taking the stairs when you can. Even if you can't walk up all sixty flights, walking five of them and then taking the elevator the rest of the way up still gives you quite a workout.

Rather than spending ten minutes circling the parking lot to find the absolutely best space available, try parking at the back of the parking lot and walking to the store. Not only will this give you exercise, but it often saves you time.

Take your dog for a much-needed walk. Getting out and enjoying the fresh air can be good for you and Fido, not to mention the added benefits to your body.

Are you the type of person who carries things to the stairs and leaves a pile to carry up later? Consider taking your belongings up the stairs every time you would normally just pile them up. Six or seven trips up the stairs throughout the day is a great way to add to your workout without stressing your time limits or lifestyle. The fringe benefit is that you do not have anything to trip over at the bottom of the stairs and it looks so clean. Just make sure you are not carrying heavy loads, following the guidelines of your particular caregiver.

Work Exercises

If you work at a desk or in an office, you might try taking a walk during a break period or lunch. Not only will it help you fit exercise in, but it will also get you out of the office and give you a chance to clear your head. Be sure to bring a change of shoes so that you are comfortable and safe when you walk.

There are also many exercises that you can do while sitting at your desk. Even when not pregnant, it is important to remember to stretch every hour while working. You can incorporate a few other simple exercises into that stretch period, which have been shown to help improve performance.

Creating Your Exercise Space

The type of exercise you do will determine, at least in part, where you will exercise. For example, walking can be done outside in the neighborhood, on a treadmill in your house, outside at a track, inside at the mall, or even inside on a track. All of these locations would be appropriate for walking.

However, it is wise always to have alternative plans in place should something come up, either weather- or life-related, that would make your location plans change. For example, in the heat of summer many avid outdoor walkers become mall walkers. It is free and air-conditioned!

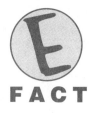

FACT

Walking clubs abound at many local area malls. Some hospitals and health centers even have clubs designed for mall walking; many are geared toward women. You might even find that some programs are pregnancy and/or new mom specific. Try calling your local mall or hospital education programs to see if there is such a walking club in your area.

Exercising at Home

If you are a person who prefers to work out in your home, there are accommodations to be made there, too. This area of your home should be a place that you can easily change into your workout area, or even better, leave as your workout area. You want a well-ventilated and open space in which to do your workouts.

Which room works best, you ask? If you occasionally do a pregnancy workout tape, you will want your space to be near a television and a VCR. If you like to see the outdoors while doing yoga, choose a spot near a window. The actual room itself is not the question, except when dealing with issues of space and practicality. Nearly any room will do.

The flooring surface might be an issue, depending on what type of exercise you choose. You might not have a choice of flooring, but you definitely want to ensure that you remove rugs that you could easily fall on or trip over, as well as pieces of furniture that are too close to the exercise area. (This does not mean moving large pieces of furniture on your own as a part of a weightlifting routine.) Know what accessories, if any, will be needed for your workout and keep them nearby.

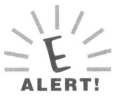

Phones, doorbells, and pagers—they all have a way of going off while you are working out. Remember that this time is your time to work out. Avoid all unnecessary interruptions for the workout period. This will help ensure a better workout and give you a much-needed break from the hustle and bustle of life.

Once you have chosen your space, remember to gather supplies before you start. There is nothing more frustrating than having to pause a tape to run to get a chair for balance, or remembering halfway through your yoga workout that you left your props in the trunk of the car. Also remember to bring your water bottle with you. You might want a towel if you perspire—anything you might need during the course of the workout.

Workout Clothes

What you wear while exercising is just as important as watching your form. The right clothing can help protect you from falls, balance problems, overheating, and dehydration. Let's not forget to mention that the right outfit can simply make you more comfortable during your workout.

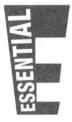

Picking the right bra is very important in pregnancy. As your breast development changes, your bra needs will be quite different. Many women experience breast changes early in the first trimester that continue throughout a pregnancy. Bra purchases are important and should not be skimped on. Find a supportive bra that prevents bouncing movements and remember that you may go through one or more bra size changes as your pregnancy progresses.

There is not one *right* type of outfit to wear, but rather choose something that keeps you comfortable, safe, and willing to exercise. When you are not pregnant and you are working out, you may have a favorite type of outfit. You might be a sweat suit type of person, or perhaps you prefer running shorts and a jogging bra. Either way, you can carry this over to pregnancy attire.

Maternity Fashion

Maternity fitness fashions are certainly becoming, well, more fashionable. Until recently, if you wanted something to work out in while pregnant, you shopped at the big and tall men's store, or from your husband's closet. Now the fashion industry has caught up with the pregnancy fitness craze.

Today's maternity wear has a variety of options for your expanding belly. Some pants offer a stretchy panel that will expand with your waist. Other garments are made as one piece and also expand as you grow. You can also find maternity wear that offers buttons to expand the width of the pant portion of your outfit. The other alternative is a stretch-band waist.

Wearing the Proper Clothing

When dressing to work out, remember to dress as you normally would, keeping in mind considerations for your pregnant body. You will probably want to wear layers of clothing, as they will allow you to remove some clothes without having to put a complete halt on your workout. With the increased blood volume circulating in your body, you might become hot more quickly.

Choose clothes that breathe. For example, cotton is great for working out and is particularly valuable in the choice of your underwear or pants. Synthetic materials in this sensitive area can make you more likely to develop a rash or even a yeast infection. While not the end of the world, this can be annoying to you and, if left untreated, such problems may cause preterm labor.

Figuring out what you need to do to maintain your current fitness level is the biggest part of getting started. You will need to talk to your practitioner and decide what types of activity are best suited for your pregnancy. Learning to add exercise into your everyday life makes it easier to become and stay fit. Ⓔ

Chapter 4
The Kegel Muscle

When you find out you are pregnant, everyone wants to share their stories with you. They seem to love to tell you horror stories about what childbirth did to their bodies. One of the favorite stories to tell is what happens to your bladder control and sex life after a baby. It does not have to be this way! You can learn exercises and information to save your sex life—and your underwear.

What Is the Kegel Muscle?

The Kegel muscle, or pubococcygeal muscle (PC), was named after Dr. Arnold Kegel. It was Dr. Kegel who identified that it was important to exercise this group of muscles. Before Dr. Kegel's work, these muscles were unheard of by the average woman.

The Anatomy

Since Dr. Kegel's discovery, we have touted the benefits of Kegel exercises to help strengthen the Kegel muscles. This hammock-like structure of muscles is located in the pelvic floor region in both men and women. In women, this muscle group actually helps hold the pelvic organs, like the bladder, in place. There are three openings to the muscle in women: the urethra, the vagina, and the anus.

Each of these openings is surrounded by a sphincter, which is comprised of voluntary and involuntary muscles. The voluntary muscles provide you with control over the release of urine and feces. The involuntary muscles hold your organs in place without you having to worry about it.

You might be thinking that this is a nice little anatomy lesson—but what does it have to do with me? The answer is simple: everything!

"Kegeling"

This little hammock of muscles can do a lot for you, with proper maintenance. "Kegeling," the act of exercising the Kegel muscle, will help you decrease the incidence of stress incontinence. *Stress incontinence* is what we call it when you cough or sneeze and wet your pants!

Kegeling can help tone the muscle to provide you with better control over the muscle group during birth. Not only will you increase your ability to push your baby out effectively, but you will also decrease the likelihood of needing an episiotomy (incision made in the perineum, area of skin between the vagina and the anus) and the likelihood of tearing.

These exercises will also help tone your pelvic floor muscles, which will result in better blood flow and will promote faster healing of this sensitive area after the birth of your baby. And the good news is that Kegel exercises are something you can do immediately post-birth.

Identifying the Kegel Muscle

You might be wondering how you are going to find this series of muscles. Put the mirror and the flashlight away! While they may help you see the area, they will not be necessary for finding the Kegel muscle.

The best advice on finding this muscle is to empty your bladder while you are going to the bathroom. After you have done so, try to imagine stopping the flow of urine. The muscles that you would contract to stop the flow of urine are the Kegel muscles.

ALERT!

Be sure that you have emptied your bladder before attempting to locate the Kegel muscle. Having urine in the bladder can potentially cause urine to back up and cause a bladder or kidney infection.

Kegeling does not have to be done only in the bathroom. Once you have learned to identify this muscle, you should not have much trouble remembering where it is located. The great news is that you can perform Kegel exercises anytime, anywhere, and no one will notice that you are doing them!

If you have trouble locating the muscles, consult your practitioner. A few women will have trouble finding them either because of poor muscle tone or medical conditions such as a prolapse of the bladder.

Improving Your Sex Life

Are you wondering what a couple of muscles that seem to have nothing to do with sex can do for your sex life? The answer is a lot. Every time you have sex, you are using the Kegel muscles. Poor vaginal tone can create a lack of sensation for you and decreased sensation for your partner.

The muscles of the vagina support the penis during intercourse and contract as you experience orgasm. A strong, well-toned muscle will provide not only more sensation for you, but your partner as well. You can even try Kegeling during intercourse. Many men report that this added sensation is very exciting. This is also a good meter of how much you are exercising. Try this test after a few weeks of Kegeling and see if your partner can tell a difference!

Sex after Baby

Eventually, when your life settles down a bit and your body has begun its recovery from the birth of your baby in earnest, you will begin to think about sex again. You might be the woman who wants to start as soon as she can, or if you are like many women, you might have a delay in your sexual desire. Both variations are normal.

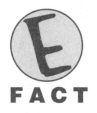

FACT

Men can Kegel, too! Yes, they too have a Kegel muscle. To do Kegels, they simply concentrate on stopping the flow of urine, or while erect, making the penis move substantially. This helps stimulate the prostate gland for health benefits of its own, including enhanced sexual pleasure.

The general guideline is that it takes about six weeks postpartum until your body is ready for sex again. There are many factors that will influence whether or not you are ready to resume physical relations with your partner. Some of these relate to the birth itself.

The Healing Process

If you had a vaginal delivery, even without any stitches, the area of the perineum will have still suffered from the trauma of giving birth. If you did have stitches, generally they will dissolve on their own in about two weeks. Your doctor or midwife will be able to give you exact details about how many stitches you had and the location of the stitches. Having sex before allowing these tissues to heal or the stitches to dissolve can result in some problems with additional trauma to the perineum and vagina.

Was your baby born by cesarean delivery? You might think that this gives you a break, and in a way it does. Unless you experienced pushing, or a vacuum or forceps were used prior to C-section, your vaginal tissues should be fairly intact. However, the waiting game is still in effect for you as well.

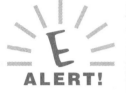

ALERT!

Doctors used to sew an extra stitch into a woman's vagina after birth. The so-called husband's stitch is no longer used and is basically an old wives' tale. Be leery of any practitioner who claims to routinely fix a problem that wasn't there before.

Risk of Infection

The main reason that you are asked to wait until your six-week postpartum checkup to resume sexual intercourse is the risk of infection. No matter how you gave birth, the site of the placenta is healing. While it is healing, your body will produce a bloody to beige-colored fluid, called *lochia*, as it heals itself. Every woman will experience this discharge after the birth of a baby.

When the lochia has stopped, the placental site has usually healed. However, it's best to wait a week or two after you stop bleeding. You might go a day or two without bleeding and assume you are healed, only to begin bleeding again a few days later. Since sex can introduce bacteria and semen into the vagina and uterus, it is wise to wait until you are completely healed before resuming intercourse.

Birth Control

Then there is the issue of birth control. Contrary to popular opinion, you can conceive again right after having a baby. This can happen even before you begin to have your periods again as ovulation can precede your first period postpartum. While it is less likely to happen to a mother who is nursing full time with no supplementation or pacifier use, it can still happen in this case, too. Therefore, it is in your best interest not to have sex without the use of birth control. Talk to your practitioner about which method is right for you and your family. Many methods are perfectly acceptable, even with breastfeeding.

Retaining Urinary Integrity

While we often tell women that having babies vaginally will wreak havoc on their urinary tracts, there are differing opinions on this statement. Some practitioners believe that having a baby vaginally is the only reason that a woman would experience problems in this area. However, problems with the Kegel muscle are present in women who have never had children or have had cesarean (surgical) births.

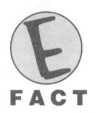

FACT

Many women have been led to believe that a vaginal birth is the main cause of urinary incontinence. However, a recent study showed that a group of nuns, who had never given birth, had the same rate of urinary incontinence as did mothers who had experienced vaginal birth.

Trouble Signs

No matter how you give birth to your baby, you can be at risk for problems. Some researchers theorize that simply being pregnant can predispose you to potential problems with urinary integrity. Some believe it is hereditary. The real issue is whether or not you have a toned Kegel muscle. This is what exercise can help provide you.

You have identified the muscle. You have started exercising. But how do you know if you are already experiencing problems with lack of muscle tone in this area? Here are some signs that will alert you to problems:

- You leak urine when you cough or sneeze.
- You leak urine with the sudden urge to urinate.
- You have already experienced a prolapse of a pelvic organ.
- You have had a previous episiotomy or vaginal surgery.

What do you do if you are already experiencing some of the symptoms of a weak muscle? The good news is that with work and exercise you can correct the problems you are already experiencing. The exercise of these muscles is so beneficial that the majority of women can fix the problem even after it has already begun, and without surgery.

Attaining Muscle Tone

There are many different ways to exercise the Kegel muscles, but before we describe the ways, remember these three easy tips:

1. Do them religiously.
2. Do them anywhere.
3. Do them for life.

The Quick Moves Exercise

The first exercise to try is "quick moves." Remember that you can do these sitting, standing, lying, or even squatting—whatever position works best for you. You can even do them in multiple settings for maximum effectiveness.

To do Kegels, simply squeeze the muscles in a set of five quick repetitions. As your muscle tone improves you can do groups of ten repetitions for a better workout. Keep repeating this Kegel exercise until you can't feel your muscles anymore or until you have reached 100 repetitions.

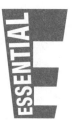

When doing your Kegels, remember that you should only be moving the muscles inside your body. If you find yourself squeezing your glutes or thighs together, you need more practice!

This simple series of quick moves will reinforce the location of the muscles. If you have previously had problems isolating them and moving only the Kegel muscles, repeated exercise will bring about better control of the area. The problem should disappear as you begin to gain strength and tone in your Kegel muscle.

The Tightening Exercise

From the quick moves exercise you will move to the next stage of Kegels, which is just a tad more involved. While tightening only your Kegel muscles, as with quick moves, you will now hold the muscle tightly for one to two seconds. Then, release the tension and repeat for a set of ten repetitions. You can build the time you flex the muscle from five to ten seconds, depending on your comfort level.

Do these tense, hold, and release Kegels at least 100 times a day. You can always do more. The goal of 100 repetitions per day should be your minimum.

The Elevator Exercise

The next step to the Kegel series is often referred to as an elevator exercise. In whatever position you choose, begin with a relaxed muscle and think of this as the first floor. Slowly tighten the muscles, as an elevator would go up to each floor, and hold the tightness as you go, increasing it slowly with each floor. When you reach the top floor of your muscle, slowly return the elevator to the first floor.

The number of floors you can add will depend on the strength of the muscle. Some women can work their way up to five, while other manage fewer. The number of floors is not as important as properly doing the exercise.

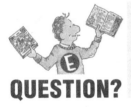

QUESTION?

How do I know if I'm doing it right?
If you are doing Kegels correctly, you will not be tightening other muscles like your buttocks or thighs. You will be isolating this internal muscle and not straining other ones in the process.

An advanced version of the elevator exercise takes your muscles on a tour of the floors with the last stop being the basement. To do this you will actually try to bulge your Kegel muscle out slightly. This should not be a harsh or forceful movement, but it will help you greatly in awareness of your body, particularly when it is time to push your baby into the world.

Reverse Kegels

Pushing is nothing more than bulging that baby's head into the bottom floor of your perineum. Some women like to think of this as a reverse Kegel. This awareness will help you be able to control the focus of your pushing phase in labor. You will have great awareness of the Kegel muscles and as you identify them during this last stage of labor, you will be able to push more effectively.

Starting slowly is the way to approach any exercise. It is the same with Kegel exercises. The more you do Kegels, the easier they are to do and the more you are able to do, not to mention you will find them becoming a habit the more often you do them.

Super Kegels

Once you have mastered the basic Kegels and have found that you are ready to move on, it's now time to try Super Kegels. Begin by tightening the Kegel muscles as tightly as you can for a count of ten and then release. Do a set of ten repetitions at least once a day.

There will be times, for personal or medical reasons, that you may wish to incorporate vaginal weights into your Kegel exercise session. Your practitioner might recommend these weights to help you increase muscle strength in the Kegel muscle.

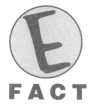

FACT

While these muscles may seem to tire very quickly and become numb, the more you exercise them, the more endurance they will develop. Kegel muscles also tend to recover very quickly from their workout.

Kegels for Life

While any exercise program you begin should be for life, the Kegel exercises are even more important for the lifelong function of your pelvic floor. You will not always know right after giving birth whether there was trauma to the area. Sometimes problems that have occurred do not even show up until you are much older. Many more women who are older suffer from the prolapse of organs like the bladder and vagina. Continuing your Kegels is the best way to prevent the need for further treatment if you have indeed suffered some trauma.

Doing Kegels as an older woman is exactly the same as when you are younger. However, some older women choose to change how they do the exercises simply to vary the routine. They can do a variety of number of repetitions; they can do a stair step or elevator type of method.

For example, squeeze the kegel muscle slightly, hold, a bit more, hold, until you get to your maximum tightness, hold again and then reverse the process until you get to the base level. As long as the muscles are being worked out, you are receiving the benefit of the exercise.

Spreading the Kegel News

Now that you know all of the amazing benefits of exercising the Kegel muscles, you might consider sharing this information with the older women in your life, like your mother and grandmother. Many older women were not given instruction on these exercises, partially because it was not known about and partially because childbirth and prenatal education was not developed as it is nowadays.

You can explain to them the benefit of the regular exercise of this muscle. You can simply instruct them how to locate the Kegel muscle. Then you can give them details on some of the exercises. You might be surprised at how much they share with you about the condition of the muscle already.

ESSENTIAL

Your grandma might have a different idea about Kegeling. Older women often feel that this exercise is "dirty" and pertains only to sex and masturbation. Trying to help educate them is important; you can help increase their health awareness.

Your Kegel muscles, while not seen, are very important. What type of obstetrical history you have will play a role in what tone you currently have in these muscles. By exercising the muscles you can improve your sex life, decrease the chance of tearing or needing an episiotomy during labor, and prevent future complications from vaginal and/or bladder prolapse. Do your Kegels for life! Ⓔ

Chapter 5

Your First Trimester

As you learn to exercise with pregnancy in mind, you will have many questions about what is and what is not appropriate. The answers to these questions will change as your body changes. Each trimester will bring new challenges to exercise. The first trimester is one of the least restrictive trimesters, but also a great time to learn about your changing body.

Exercise Barriers in the First Trimester

The first trimester, as with each trimester, brings about interesting situations in which you must learn to maneuver in order to exercise. Adjusting to the news of the pregnancy and the rapid body changes are the biggest hurdles to overcome in early pregnancy exercise.

For some women, the early stages of pregnancy do not bring many physical changes to their lifestyles, particularly if the pregnancy was planned and you have been "acting pregnant" during the preconception phase. The news of your pregnancy may still come as a shock, even though you were trying to conceive. This shocked phase of pregnancy is real for everyone and can hamper your efforts to exercise. Reminding yourself that pregnancy is a natural process will help with this feeling.

Though they will vary from woman to woman, the physical symptoms of pregnancy—from morning sickness to fatigue—are usually not noticed until about six weeks from the last menstrual period. For those who experience physical symptoms, adjusting to them can be the hardest part of exercising in the early days of pregnancy.

Morning Sickness

The one thing that most women expect from early pregnancy is nausea and vomiting, commonly referred to as morning sickness. Anyone who has been pregnant will tell you that this term is a misnomer, because it can strike at any time of the day or night, sometimes all of the above. Clearly, morning sickness can get in the way of your feeling well enough to exercise. Try eating a bit of protein, staying well hydrated, and exercising to the point of comfort. Some women say that exercise actually helps them avoid some feelings of nausea.

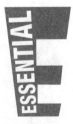

Early pregnancy nausea that is extreme, called *hyperemesis gravidarum*, may be a really good reason not to exercise. If you experience this, you may have trouble ingesting enough calories to gain weight, and dehydration is common. Expending more calories while exercising may not be right at this point, nor is it wise to run the risk of dehydration. Save exercise for later.

Combating nausea and/or vomiting can encompass a lot of friendly advice. Many of the tricks that have worked for other women will help you, but obviously everyone will respond differently. Try some of the things you hear women talking about and ignore the ones that do not fit your beliefs or lifestyle. Here is a small sample of some remedies to try:

- Crackers before you get out of bed
- Flat sodas or colas
- Lemonade or lemon candy
- Ginger tea, snaps, or candy
- Snack before bed to avoid low blood sugar
- Ice water (sipping slowly)
- Small, frequent meals

If you find yourself feeling queasy only at certain points of the day or night, try to rearrange your exercise schedule for a time when you are feeling less ill. This might mean switching the type of exercise you do for a while, but again consistency is key in exercising.

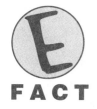

A pregnant exerciser may be concerned about the risks of miscarriage because of the exercise she does during early pregnancy. However, studies have shown that the rate of miscarriage is the same for those who exercise as for those who do not, about 16 to 17 percent in both groups.

Fatigue, Insomnia, and Fear

Fatigue is often talked about among newly pregnant women as one of the most surprising and hardest to deal with physical symptoms. While you might have expected some of the other physical symptoms, the feeling of utter exhaustion is completely unexpected for some women. If you find early pregnancy draining all of your energy, you are not alone. The good news is that there are ways to combat these symptoms.

Exercise is probably one of the better ways to deal with the fatigue of early pregnancy, yet it might not seem like the solution. After all, how will expending even more energy help you with being dead-dog tired? The answer is simple: Exercise helps your body run more efficiently, helps you sleep better at night, and generally improves your physical and mental well-being.

In addition to fatigue, some women suffer from insomnia. This can come in the form of either having difficulty falling asleep or awakening early and being unable to get back to sleep. Avoiding stimulants like caffeine can be a big help in combating excessive wakefulness or insomnia. Also avoid napping during the day. Remember to exercise during the day or very early evening and not just before bedtime. If you exercise just before bed, it may be harder to fall asleep as it does stimulate the body for a period of time, whereas exercise earlier in the day will actually help you sleep better at night.

Another exercise stopper to avoid is fear. Many women are fearful that exercising while pregnant will cause birth defects or other problems with their pregnancy. Some think that a pregnant body is not meant to handle the strain of exercise or the intensity that may come along with exercise. Education is the key to overcoming a fear of exercise while pregnant.

Special Considerations

How much or how often you exercise during your pregnancy will largely be determined by your pregnancy history, as well as other factors such as your current fitness level. If you have had problems with preterm labor or other difficulties in a previous pregnancy, it is very important to discuss this with your doctor or midwife. While this may not affect your current pregnancy at all, more monitoring is generally indicated.

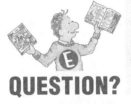

QUESTION?

How will I know if I should stop exercising?
If you experience any pain, bleeding, excessive fatigue, dizziness, or any other symptom that concerns you, stop and talk to your practitioner before resuming exercise.

Keeping an eye on the signs and signals your body is sending you during this pregnancy will help you avoid certain problems. By listening, you and your practitioner can learn to tell when changes are going on that may indicate early labor, poor fetal growth, and other complications. These complications are not always predictable in pregnancy. However, if you experienced these problems in a previous pregnancy you might be at a higher risk for a repeated scenario.

Your current fitness level will play a large part in how you are able to handle exercise in this pregnancy. If you have previously been fit and have recently seen a decline in your fitness levels, this can be disappointing. Remember that pregnancy is a time of maintaining health and wellness, not of building yourself up into a newly buff body.

Improving Your Posture

You probably have not had a lecture on proper posture since you were about thirteen years old. However, the importance of posture goes way beyond what your mother and grandmother lectured about. How you hold your body will help you stay comfortable and help you deal with pregnancy discomforts in a much easier manner. Imagine your body as a building, and proper posture is the foundation. If your body is built on a shaky foundation, it would fall under the added pressure of changes to its structure, like the added weight and movement of the uterus and baby during pregnancy.

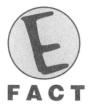

FACT

During pregnancy, you actually have a decrease in the synovial fluid in your joints. This makes them more prone to injury. Be sure to avoid bouncy and jerking motions while exercising.

During pregnancy you must continually adjust how you hold yourself and carry yourself. Your center of gravity, which is located just below the umbilicus (belly button), will also shift as your uterus and baby grow, usually starting in the fourth month, or sixteen to eighteen weeks. To prevent improper posture from becoming a habit, you really need to watch how you stand, sit, and carry yourself during the months of pregnancy.

The benefits of maintaining proper body posture during pregnancy are many, including:

- Fewer backaches
- Better body awareness
- Ease in breathing difficulties

Posture goes beyond just standing up "straight," particularly when you consider your spine is not a straight series of bones, but rather a series of S-curved bones. You want to ensure that you hold your shoulders back, and your feet are shoulder-width apart. Tuck in your tailbone and tuck in your chin so that the top of your head (the crown) is up. This means holding your head as if a string were pulling at the top and holding the shoulders back while your pelvis is loose and mobile.

This might feel odd to you at first, but with practice it will become a habit. Some women find that having friends and family remind them works well, while others place stickers in appropriate places to remind them to stand up straight!

ESSENTIAL

When getting up from a sitting or sleeping position, remember to use proper body mechanics. Try to assume a kneeling position and bring one foot forward and push your body up. Use the bed or a chair for support as you do this. This will help you prevent injury and maintain safety.

Sitting

When sitting, it is possible to avoid slumping over the desk at work, slouching in your chair, or even in the car. Remember to sit on your "sit bones," the ischial tuberosities. They will bear the weight of your body. Place your hands on your knees and pull yourself into an upright position. You will feel your spine lengthen. Remember to tuck your chin in and pull your crown up, as you would with standing postures. If you need some help keeping your pelvis tucked in, consider sitting with a towel tucked under your sit bones.

Standing

Standing tall is not the only solution to a standing situation. Many women find themselves in situations where they stand for long periods of time. While standing "straight" and with the proper posture, you will avoid problems such as backache. There are things that you can do to make this situation more comfortable.

If you will be standing in one location, like a workstation, for long periods of time, try moving around whenever possible. Be sure to stand with your feet shoulder-width apart. Shifting your weight from leg to leg can help with the stress and strain. Wearing low or no heels is also important. Some women find that placing a box or a telephone book under the desk or table and propping a foot up also reduces strain on their bodies. If these methods do not help you solve your body aches, see if it is possible to obtain a very tall chair to place at your workstation. When all else fails, ask your practitioner for recommendations for the workstation, as sometimes employers need some medical prodding.

Lifting and Bending

When lifting something or bending, it is also wise to watch your body. You probably bend over more often than you think as you pick things up around the house, or lift a child into the bathtub. However, even reaching above your head to grab something off a tall shelf can pose a potential hazard to body mechanics. Remember to keep your chin and pelvis tucked, do not let your knees go beyond your toes, and bend at the knees. Never bend at the waist, this can unduly strain your back, not to mention that in the coming months your waist will be disappearing!

Sleeping

Most of us regard bedtime as a time to flop on the bed and crash. You find that when you are pregnant, life is not so simple, nor is how you sleep. Remember that sleeping in a good position will help you get more sleep down the road. During this first trimester, your sleeping arrangements will not be altered much, except by increased middle-of-the-night trips to the bathroom. Continue to pay attention to your sleeping situation as the months go by and your pregnant abdomen begins to swell.

ALERT!

Avoid dehydration at all costs! Drink water every chance you get—before, during, and after a workout. Severe dehydration can cause major problems like preterm labor, but even mild dehydration can lead to problems like headaches, poor concentration abilities, and fatigue. Your body needs about 48 to 64 ounces of water every day, and even more when exercising.

Easing into the Groove

Don't let pregnancy scare you away from exercising. Even if you have never really been a dedicated exercise person, there are ways to exercise in pregnancy. Remember that the benefits of even mild exercise are many to you and your baby.

Some women choose to wait until the end of their first trimester to begin exercising, though there is no real reason to do so if you are only experiencing normal first trimester symptoms. In fact, there are many references out there that point to exercise as a way to relieve some of the problems like nausea, fatigue, and dietary concerns. The key to the appropriate amount of exercise in the first trimester, particularly for those who have not exercised before, is to avoid overdoing it. Remember to let your body be your guide.

Start with easy exercises for beginners, like simple exercise routines. Walking or swimming, for example, can be continued throughout pregnancy and offers numerous benefits. Even bicycling, stationary or regular, can be continued for much of pregnancy. Try creating your own routine that fulfills your needs for exercise while enhancing your body's ability to gestate.

One of the biggest problems for women beginning exercise is sticking with their choice of activities. Remember that sporadic exercise can be worse for you than no exercise at all. So find a plan that works well for you, your body, and your baby.

Exercises for the First Trimester

During the beginning part of pregnancy there are very few exercises that you must avoid. Because your uterus is not very big, you do not have some of the special concerns that you will have in later parts of pregnancy and you still have a lot of mobility.

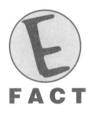

FACT

Keeping exercise logs of your workouts is a great way to keep yourself motivated, not to mention to see how far you have come. Do not hesitate to bring your exercise logs in to show your practitioner. He or she will be glad to know you are taking such an interest in your health.

The main point to focus on would be to watch how you are exercising. Practicing good posture will help keep you and your baby safe while allowing you a good workout. Be sure to watch for signs of problems while exercising, particularly temperature- and dehydration-related concerns. Overheating is actually a bigger hazard in early pregnancy than it is in the second and third trimester. If your body becomes too warm, so might your baby. During the first trimester, all of your baby's major organ systems are forming, making it more susceptible to minute changes in the body. This is not as much of a concern when you are an experienced exerciser.

Other than these few simple precautions, your exercise limitations in the first trimester will be the same ones you would normally avoid. Anything that your body responds negatively to while you exercise is also contraindicated.

Warmups

Just as a good warmup is important during exercise prior to pregnancy, it is probably more important during pregnancy because of the physical changes that are taking place. The first trimester is an odd time because you don't really "feel" pregnant yet. Your body certainly isn't showing many outward signs of the good news, and you may find yourself forgetting that you're pregnant.

A proper warmup should last at least five to ten minutes. The goal of the warmup is to prepare your body for a workout by stretching your muscles and getting your heart pumping. The type of warmup you choose, will depend, in part, on what exercise you do. By getting into the habit of a good warmup during the first trimester, the benefits of this brief but all-important time will become even more important during the second and third trimesters of pregnancy.

Again, one of the reasons that the warmup period is so important during pregnancy is that your body is producing hormones, like relaxin, which actually make your ligaments, tendons, and joints looser. This is to aid in the birth process. For purposes of exercise, this means that you need to have extra caution about exercising and protecting these areas. A warmup is one step in this protection process.

ESSENTIAL

Watch your salt intake! Do not limit your salt intake for fear of swelling; this can actually have the opposite effect. Your body needs salt. Try salting your food to taste as opposed to avoiding salt or overdoing it.

Cool-downs

Cooling down is another important aspect of every workout. It is hard on any of us to abruptly stop one activity and begin another activity. Your body is no different in this respect. The purpose of the cool-down is to gradually reduce your heart rate back to your baseline. This time also encourages your muscles to cool down.

Use the cool-down period to lead into a brief relaxation period for your mind if this works for you. Not only will you receive the physical benefits of exercise, but the mental exercises will help place you in a greater state of relaxation. The further you are in your pregnancy the more benefit you will see from this practice.

Sample Exercise Program

The exercises listed here are generally fine for the first trimester of pregnancy. Remember to modify any exercises that you need to, and skip those that cause pain. Show these exercises to your doctor or midwife if you have any questions about the exercises themselves or your ability to participate in these exercises.

Warmup

Try all of these exercises or a combination of them for your warmup:

■ Neck Stretch

Stand with your feet shoulder-width apart. Let your shoulders be held up and back. The crown of your head should be pulling upward. Slowly let your chin drop to your chest and hold it there for five to ten seconds. Return your head to the neutral position. Gently let your chin drop to your chest again, and slowly roll your head toward your left shoulder, again holding it for five to ten seconds. Repeat this with your right side. It is okay if you can't hold your head all the way down. Move until you feel the stretch, but not pain. Do this series three to five times.

■ Shoulder Rounds

Without changing the position of your body, try to exaggerate a shrug upward with your shoulders, bringing them to your ears. Hold this position for five to ten seconds. Then relax your shoulders back to their beginning position. Move your shoulders in small circles forward for ten repetitions, and then reverse and go backward for ten repetitions.

Wrist/Ankle Rotations

While holding your body in its correct posture, extend your arms in front of you. They should be at your chest level, just below your shoulder. Rotate your wrists forward and backward, about ten small circles each direction. Repeat the same exercise with your ankles.

Hip Rotations

This is a lot of fun! Stand with your feet shoulder-width apart and tuck your pelvis in; think of flattening your back. Begin to sway your hips in a clockwise motion, about ten circles. Stop and repeat in a counter-clockwise motion. It looks a lot like belly-dancing!

Standing Exercises

Wall Pushups

Facing the wall, place your hands palm down on the wall; walk your feet backward, away from the wall (see **FIGURE 5-1**). Slowly bend your elbows,

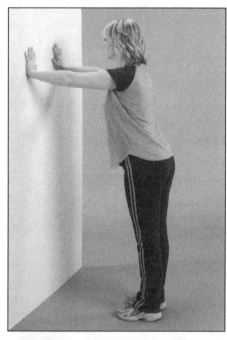

FIGURE 5-1
Wall Pushups, starting position.
Watch your posture!

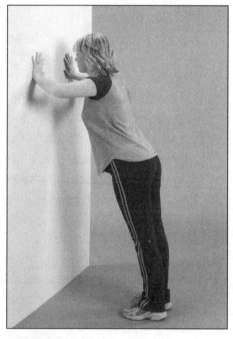

FIGURE 5-2
Wall Pushups, bent elbows position

bringing your upper body closer to the wall. Hold this position for three to ten seconds (see **FIGURE 5-2**). Do about ten repetitions of the exercise. Remember to keep your spine in the proper alignment while doing this exercise.

■ Posture Retraining

Place your back against the wall; slowly walk your feet forward until they are 6 to 8 inches in front of you. Press your glutes, shoulder blades, and the back of your head into the wall (see **FIGURE 5-3**). Slowly raise your arms at a 90-degree angle, bent elbow to the wall, and press them to the wall as well. Slowly raise your arms, keeping them on the wall, above your head (see **FIGURE 5-4**).

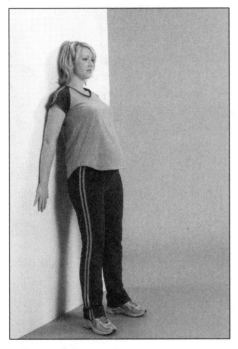

FIGURE 5-3
Posture Retraining

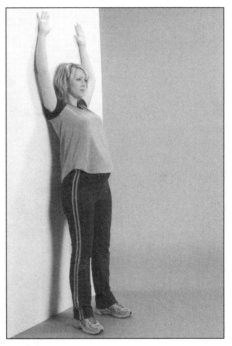

FIGURE 5-4
Enjoy a good stretch and feel the benefits of proper posture.

Lunge

Stand up without the support of the wall and step back with your left leg. Your upper body should remain facing forward and not moving. Be sure to keep your right knee above your right ankle, as leaning or twisting could cause injury (see **FIGURE 5-5**). Lower your body until your right thigh is nearly parallel to the floor. Raise your body by pressing into your right foot (see **FIGURE 5-6**). Do about ten repetitions of this exercise and then repeat on the opposite side.

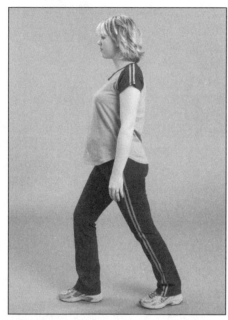

FIGURE 5-5
Lunge

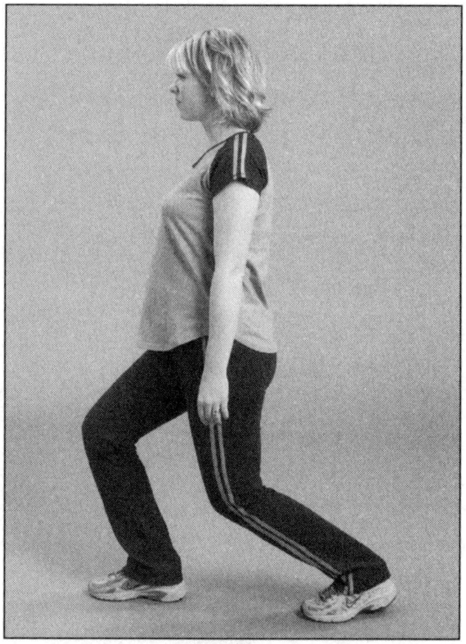

FIGURE 5-6
Lunge, with right thigh almost parallel to the floor

Heel Raises

Lean on a wall, facing the wall. Hold the wall with the palms of your hands. Extend your feet, raising your heels, like standing on the tip of your toes.

Sitting and Lying Exercises

Tailor Sit

This is one that can be done while reading on the floor, or at any time. Basically, it's sitting as you did in kindergarten, cross-legged. For every opportunity you have to sit on the floor, do this exercise.

■ Pelvic Rock/Pelvic Tilt

This is the perfect exercise for backaches in pregnancy. It will not only help prevent them but cure them as well. Assume an all-fours position, down on your hands and knees. Think of holding your back in its natural alignment (see **FIGURE 5-7**). Then, tuck only your pelvis in, bringing your pubic bone toward your neck. Be sure to move only your pelvis (see **FIGURE 5-8**). If it helps, have someone hold your pelvis so that you can learn to isolate this area. Later, this exercise can be done in different positions. You need to do two sets of twenty repetitions of the pelvic tilts. For an added bonus, do another set of twenty repetitions just before bed to help you sleep.

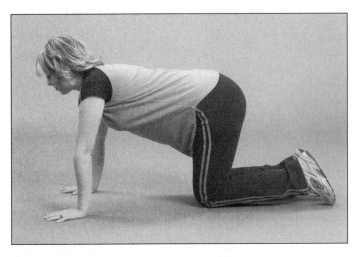

FIGURE 5-7
Pelvic Rock/
Pelvic Tilt

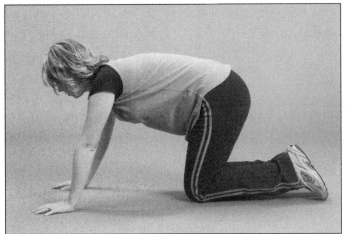

FIGURE 5-8
Be sure to avoid simply rounding your back. Feel the stretch in your lower back and pelvis.

■ Squat

This can help strengthen the muscles of your thighs to allow for an easier time at birth, if you choose to give birth in this position. Start by using a chair or a partner and stand facing it/him/her with your feet shoulder-width apart. Slowly lower your body, as he lowers his. Gently go down, while keeping your heels on the floor (see **FIGURE 5-9**). You will probably require some practice doing this exercise until you can do it alone and go down into a near-sitting position. Do ten squats, holding each one five to ten seconds. Avoid bouncing in between squats.

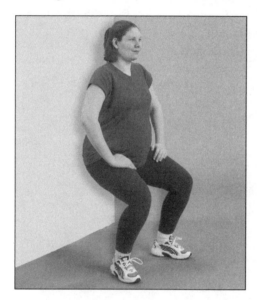

FIGURE 5-9
The Squat is great for stretching your inner thighs and preparing for labor.

■ Neck Roll-ups

Lie on the floor on your back as flat as you can. Tilt your pelvis up, so that your spine is flat on the floor. Slowly begin to curl your body up from the chin to the neck, bringing your head with your chin. Pull up until your shoulder blades are off the floor (see **FIGURE 5-10**). Hold this pose for five to ten seconds. Repeat ten times.

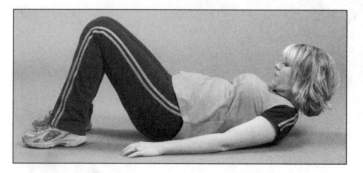

FIGURE 5-10
The Neck Roll-up will help strengthen your neck and stretch it to relieve tension.

■ Hip Abduction Lying

Lie on your back with your knees bent, feet flat on the floor, and your shoulders and hips firmly on the floor. Place your right ankle on your left knee. Bring your left knee toward your chest by grabbing your left thigh with your left hand (see **FIGURE 5-11**). Hold this for about five seconds. Repeat on the opposite side.

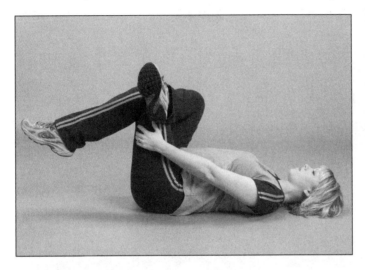

FIGURE 5-11
Hip Abduction Lying provides a good stretch of the hip muscles, which become tense and sore in pregnancy.

■ Child's Pose

Kneel on the floor, separating your knees slightly. Put your big toes together and sit back with your buttocks on the heels of your feet. Stretch your arms over your head (see **FIGURE 5-12**). Hold this pose for five seconds, releasing a bit more with each breath. If this reach is too far for you as a beginner or later in pregnancy, let your elbows rest on your forearms to alleviate some of the tension.

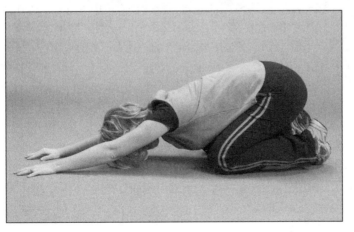

FIGURE 5-12
The Child's Pose is great for providing the stretch of the back so desperately needed in pregnancy.

■ Cat Pose

Get on your hands and knees on the floor with your spine straight, not bowed. As you exhale, lift your right arm and left leg, extending each, as you think about contracting the muscles in the raised arm and in your glutes (see **FIGURE 5-13**). Hold this pose for up to five seconds, releasing it on an exhale breath. Return to the starting position and repeat using your opposite limbs.

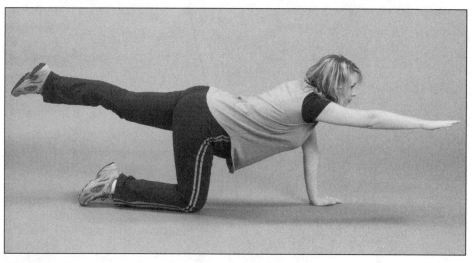

FIGURE 5-13
The Cat Pose

Cool-down

Many people simply do the their warmup for their cool-down. However, you can add more exercises to this section, because your body is already stretched and warmed up. Remember, the goal is to bring your body down slowly from its excited exercise state. Ending your cool-down with mental relaxation is important as well. Consider doing more pelvic tilts, as well as going through the entire stretching motions. To this add:

■ Full Body Extension

Lying on your back, extend your arms above your head and lengthen your legs, much like the side lying extension. Hold this pose for ten seconds and repeat. You can then choose a position for relaxation.

■ Side Lying Stretches

Lying on your right side, stretch your right arm over your body as if reaching for something above your head. Focus on extending the arm as well at the leg and body (see **FIGURE 5-14**). This should feel like a good tension release. Hold this pose for about ten seconds. Repeat on the left side.

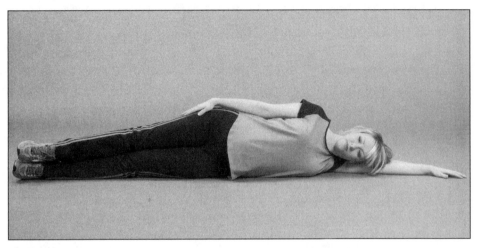

FIGURE 5-14
Side Lying Stretches are great for releasing tension in the entire body.

Relaxation

Just as you must exercise your body to prepare for pregnancy, labor, and parenthood, exercising the mind is also important. Relaxation is a vital part of your exercise program. After working out your body, your mind is in a prime state to do relaxation. It also helps promote relaxation of the body and the cooling down period.

There are three basic types of relaxation: physical, mental, and emotional. Physical relaxation is simply the release of tension from the muscles of your body. Certain positions will help promote this type of relaxation. The best positions do not allow one body part to rest upon another. This prevents you from adding tension to your body.

Mental relaxation is simply clearing your mind of extra thoughts. By allowing your mind to ease itself into a relaxed state, you can train yourself to achieve this feeling of peace during even the most stressful situations.

Emotional relaxation comes with easing the mind and clearing the thoughts of everyday life. This allows your mind to bring to the surface issues that are bothersome to you and determine a solution for them. This might be done in a dream state or in a period of deep relaxation. Allowing your fears and concerns to surface allows you to address these issues before they can add more stress and tension to your life.

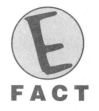

FACT

Women who practice relaxation techniques in pregnancy tend to be able to cope with labor more quickly and efficiently than their non-practicing counterparts. Remember this when you think about skipping a session!

Learning to Relax

Your body can benefit greatly from learning how to relax. Once you are in labor, it is a last-ditch effort to try to learn these skills. The benefits of relaxation can be seen, particularly if you have been practicing during your pregnancy. You find that you are more able to let the muscles of your body—namely, your uterus—do its work of contracting, without adding tension to the mix of labor. The ability to use mental images can help transport you to another place during labor, thus reducing the amount of stress hormones circulating through your body during the birth process. You will generally feel a sense of well-being as you relax and let your body do its work.

The Side Lying Position

A side lying position for relaxation is easiest to assume and is appropriate for all trimesters. Using pillows will help you achieve maximum comfort, even if your belly has not started expanding yet. Place one pillow under your head and lie on your side. Either side is fine, though some people have a preference. One hand is placed behind your body and one hand in front (see **FIGURE 5-15**). You should not place your hands under your body or your pillow. Use the other pillow to prop up your leg from the knee to the ankle, making sure that all your joints are supported. The bottom leg should be gently laid behind you.

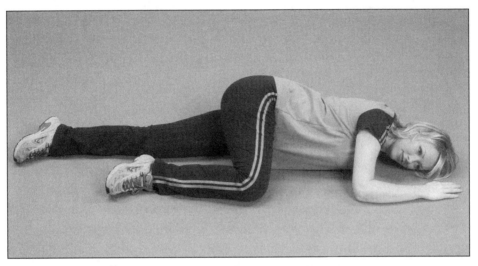

FIGURE 5-15
Use the Side Lying Position for comfort during relaxation or sleep during pregnancy.

Tense-Release Relaxation

One of the first relaxations you can learn is called a *tense-release relaxation*. All you do is mentally work your way down your body and tense each muscle you think of and then deliberately release it. This allows you to learn what tension feels like in your body. Start with your head, and work your way to your feet. You can also do this exercise with your partner.

Remember to keep your muscles relaxed after you have done the tension exercise with each group. Common problem areas are the jaw, the forehead, and your shoulders. Try to sink into your pillows and deliberately relax your face and let your jaw fall open. If you are holding up any part of your body, you need to physically stop and concentrate on relaxing that area.

Visualization

Visualization is another relaxation tool for you to use. This tool will not work for everyone, but remember that you do not have to use a script or any other prop. This should be something that works for you. You might choose to relive a certain moment in your life, for example, a great vacation or a romantic moment. Focusing on the baby is one way to help center yourself during this relaxation period. You might try imagining how your baby is growing this week, and watch, through your mind's eye, the development and progress of your little one.

Finding Time to Relax

Relaxation need not take a long time to do. A key thing to remember is that the more you practice the less time it can take. Try to fit in at least two practice sessions a day and one preferably with your husband or labor coach. This will begin the preparation for birth.

The first trimester can be a difficult time to exercise. Your body is undergoing so many changes and learning to deal with nausea and fatigue can make exercise much more difficult. As you ease into a routine, it will become easier. Learn which exercises you can and cannot do and be sure to find time for relaxation along the way to aid in the mental parts of pregnancy. (E)

Chapter 6

Your Second Trimester

Often referred to as the honeymoon phase of pregnancy, your second trimester is usually one of great well-being. You might feel as if you have more energy. You are probably starting to show a bit, making your pregnancy seem a bit more real. Use this time to continue your fitness training to prolong this feeling of well-being.

Exercise Barriers in the Second Trimester

Unlike your first trimester when nausea, vomiting, and fatigue reigned supreme, your second trimester is probably less exhausting. In fact, most women find this to be the best phase of pregnancy. Don't be concerned if you wouldn't quite put it that way. Remember, the range of normal varies widely.

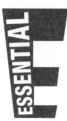

Even if you're feeling and looking great in this second part of pregnancy, there may be reasons to stop or modify your exercise routine. Generally, your doctor or midwife will discuss this need with you, but you should always feel comfortable bringing the subject up with him or her, or cutting back on your own.

Placenta Previa

As previously discussed, placenta previa is a condition in which the placenta covers all or part of the cervix. This actually comes in degrees from a full previa, where the entire cervix is covered by the placenta, to a marginal or partial previa, where only part of the cervix is covered. You might be diagnosed with a previa if you have bleeding or a mid-trimester ultrasound.

The good news is that over 95 percent of all placenta previas will naturally resolve themselves without you ever lifting a finger. The reason this happens is that the lower segment of the uterus does much of its growth in the latter half of the second trimester and in the third trimester. When this growth occurs, the placenta "moves" away from the cervix resolving the problem.

If the placenta previa does not resolve itself by the end of pregnancy, a cesarean section is planned. A baby cannot be born through the placenta. If labor begins, bleeding may endanger you or the baby due to blood loss.

When it comes to exercise, your restrictions will depend largely on the extent of your previa and whether or not you've had any bleeding. If you have an appointment for an ultrasound and are told about the previa, discontinue all exercise until you talk to your doctor or midwife about the safety of resuming exercise.

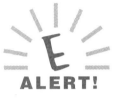

ALERT!

In this part of pregnancy, you will see a dramatic increase in your blood volume. If you have your blood tested for anemia at this juncture, you might be given a false diagnosis of anemia, because it takes the red blood cells a bit to catch up with their production. Never hesitate to ask to be retested.

Anemia

Anemia is also known as iron deficiency. Many pregnant women have this very common problem. It is mostly likely to be diagnosed in the second trimester of pregnancy because of routine blood work done at your practitioner's office. Your red blood cells act as your body's oxygen-carrying messengers in your blood. Pregnancy demands more oxygen because you need oxygen for your baby as well as for your normal needs. When you are anemic, this ability is decreased.

Signs of anemia include:

- Fatigue
- Shortness of breath
- Paleness
- Loss of energy
- Weakness
- Low blood pressure

Even if your doctor or midwife doesn't test your blood for anemia, be sure to report these symptoms at your visits. While you may put it off as being just another part of pregnancy, anemia is something that can greatly impact you, even at the time of birth. You don't wish to take the risks associated with anemia when they can be easily treated, usually with just some minor dietary changes.

If you are anemic, you may need to back down on your exercise levels a bit. As you can see, the symptoms of anemia would make it difficult to exercise anyway. As you build your iron stores back up, and as your iron levels rise and become less affected by anemia, you can gradually increase your workouts.

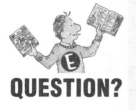

What about prenatal vitamins?
Prenatal vitamins can't provide you with everything you need. In fact, much of the iron you take in your vitamin form will not be absorbed. Try eating foods rich in iron, such as dark green leafy vegetables, red meats, and some fortified cereals. Never depend solely on a vitamin for your nutrition needs.

Preterm Labor

As opposed to late miscarriage, which is technically defined by many states as either a specific gestation, or a specific fetal weight, no matter the condition of the baby at birth, preterm labor is defined as any labor or series of contractions that occur before thirty-seven weeks' gestation (from your last menstrual period). The risk of preterm labor is that if your baby is born before it is ready, it can suffer severe health consequences, including many that are life-threatening. Your doctor or midwife should discuss with you how to be aware of signs of preterm labor and what the procedures are for calling in if you think you're in early labor.

Signs of preterm labor to watch for include:

- Dull, low backache.
- Increase in vaginal discharge.
- Bleeding from the vagina.
- Sudden gush of fluid from the vagina (waters breaking).
- Slow, continuous trickle of fluid from the vagina.
- Four or more contractions an hour.
- Increase in vaginal or pelvic pressure.
- Decrease in fetal movement.
- Feeling that something's not right.

Call your practitioner right away if you experience any of these signs of early labor. Your doctor or midwife might warn you about some other specific signs, so be sure to add these to your list and know what to do if you experience them. Don't let anyone put you off, or your fear of bothering someone stop you from making the call.

If you experience preterm labor, it is important to follow your practitioner's instructions to the letter. This will probably include limiting your ability to exercise. He or she may even order bed rest for you either at home or in the hospital. Either way exercise at this point in pregnancy would be more detrimental to your health and well-being and that of your baby. Be sure to ask any questions you have of your doctor or midwife. These are obviously not the only reasons to modify your workouts. Always talk to your doctor or midwife at each visit about your routines and how you are modifying them as your pregnancy progresses.

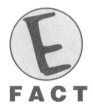

FACT

Prematurity is the leading cause of death and illness in newborn babies. With proper treatment and early awareness, oftentimes preterm labor can be stopped, thus preventing the early birth of your baby.

Special Considerations

If your practitioner has cleared you for exercise during this pregnancy, there are still some body changes that you need to be aware of before you work out. Again, you may be feeling the best you've felt all pregnancy, but keeping these body changes in mind will help alleviate potential injuries down the road.

Center of Gravity

During the second trimester, your center of gravity will begin to switch. It's something so subtle you are unlikely to detect much of anything. However, some women do report feeling a bit more clumsy at this point than before they became pregnant.

This is the time to give up high heels, walking on stilts, and anything else you might do that requires a lot of balance. For your exercise routines, this will mean you need to be constantly aware of your footing. Wear sensible shoes to avoid slipping and falling.

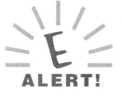

ALERT!

Do not exercise in stocking feet, or even walk around the house if you can help it. Always use the hand-rails when you take the stairs. Use good body mechanics when getting up or down from sitting or lying positions. This is particularly true of places where falls are more likely, such as the pool or bathtub.

Lying on Your Back

It was a long-held belief that pregnant women should not lie on their backs after the sixteenth week of pregnancy. The theory behind this was that after this point in pregnancy, the uterus was so large that lying on your back decreased the blood flow from the vena cava (the main vein running down your posterior side) to the uterus and your baby, also lowering your blood pressure and affecting blood flow return from your legs.

This condition, called *maternal supine hypotension syndrome*, was never truly studied until recently. When the studies were done, it was found that many women didn't actually experience any of the symptoms of complications. This has led the medical world to believe that short periods of exercise on the back during the latter trimesters are perfectly acceptable if you do not suffer from maternal supine hypotension syndrome.

Signs for maternal supine hypertension syndrome include:

- Dizziness
- Shortness of breath
- Passing out (extremely rare)

If you experience any of these while lying on your back, simply roll to your side until you feel you have recovered.

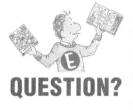

QUESTION?

Does sleeping on my back put my baby at risk?
Maternal supine hypotension syndrome can occur while sleeping on your back. The good news is that most of the time, you would wake up upon feeling these symptoms, even in your sleep. Generally, you're not even aware of why you awoke; you just naturally change positions and go back to sleep.

Enjoying Your Renewed Energy

The changes in the second trimester can be quite dramatic. You might wake up one morning and feel like a cloud has been lifted. You may not even feel very pregnant in the classic sense of nausea and grouchiness. This is the trimester when you begin to wear maternity clothes and begin to feel your baby move. What's not to feel great about?

Be sure to take advantage of this pregnancy period. Use the time to get out and enjoy life. Take more walks; spend more time doing things you enjoy. Simply enjoy the pregnancy.

Exercises for the Second Trimester

During the first part of the second trimester, you won't notice much difference in how you need to do your exercises. As the trimester progresses, and your abdomen begins to expand, you will notice changes that you need to make for comfort and safety. Things to watch for include proper clothing and ventilation to avoid overheating. To stay well hydrated, it might take more water than the previous trimester. And general safety issues, like the shift in the center of gravity, should be noted.

Warmups and Cool-downs

You learned about what constitutes a proper warmup in the previous chapter. The warmup is no less important the more exercise experience you have. Pregnancy makes this particularly true.

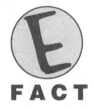

ALERT!

During the second trimester, you may be lulled into a false sense of security because the pregnancy is "old news"—and besides, you feel great! Don't let this type of attitude keep you from warming up. Remember, those hormones can add injury to insult if you do have a problem.

The cool-down period is still a signal to your body that your workout is over. It's also a time for an important mental shift to take place so you can gradually begin to be aware of changes in your body. The cool-down helps protect your muscles and prevent injury. There is never an appropriate time to skip the cool-down.

Relaxation

If you've started childbirth or relaxation classes, this would be the time to try to incorporate some of your teachings into your workout. You can do some self-relaxation at the end of each cool-down period to entice your mind and to relax your body.

FACT

Childbirth classes come in many different varieties. Choose one that is independently taught by a certified instructor. There are many organizations to choose from: Lamaze (*www.lamaze-childbirth.com*); ICEA (*www.icea.org*); and the Bradley Method (*www.bradleybirth.com*). Learn about the different philosophies and find an instructor in your area.

Progressive relaxation is one great tool to use in life and in labor. Find a comfortable position for relaxing, like side lying or semi-sitting. Beginning at the top of your head, imagine yourself releasing tension from the top of your head as you exhale. Slowly go down through all the major parts of your body, paying particular attention to your personal trouble spots for tension. Make sure to include your forehead, jaw, neck, shoulders, arms, wrists, hands, abdomen, upper and lower back, pelvis, pelvic floor, thighs, buttocks, calves, and feet. Feel free to include other parts, or even do fingers and toes individually.

Sample Exercise Program

The exercises listed here are generally fine for the second trimester of pregnancy. Remember to modify any exercises that you need to modify and skip those that cause pain. Show these exercises to your doctor or midwife if you have any questions about the exercises themselves, or your ability to participate in the exercises.

Warmup

Try all of these exercises or a combination of them for your warmup. For variations on these warmup exercises, try some of them on your birth ball.

■ Neck Stretch

Stand with your feet shoulder-width apart. Let your shoulders be held up and back. The crown of your head should be pulling upward. Slowly, let your chin drop to your chest and hold it there for five to ten seconds. Return your head to the neutral position. Slowly, let your left ear rest on your left shoulder, again holding it for five to ten seconds. Repeat this to your right side. It is okay if you can't hold your head all the way down. Move until you feel the stretch, but without pain. Do this series three to five times.

■ Wrist/Ankle Rotations

While holding your body in its correct posture, extend your arms in front of you. They should be at your chest level, just below your shoulder. Rotate your wrists forward and backward, about ten small circles each direction. Repeat the same exercise with your ankles.

■ Hip Rotations

This is a lot of fun! Stand with your feet shoulder-width apart and tuck your pelvis in; think of flattening your back. Begin to sway your hips in a clockwise motion, about ten circles. Stop and repeat in a counter-clockwise motion. It looks a lot like belly-dancing!

■ Knee Bends

Stand with your feet slightly greater than shoulder-width apart. Begin by tilting your pelvis and begin to bend your knees. Keep your head remaining upright and don't move your feet on the floor. Go down as far as comfortable, without compromising your balance. Return to your original pose. This is a slow motion. Do not jerk or bounce. Repeat this exercise for a total of ten repetitions.

■ Knee Raises

Stand with your feet slightly greater than shoulder-width apart, placing your hands on your hips or at your sides (see **FIGURE 6-1**). While maintaining your proper posture, lift your right knee until it is at about a 90-degree angle (see **FIGURE 6-2**). Slowly lower your leg to its beginning position. Repeat this exercise for a total of ten repetitions and then switch knees for another ten repetitions. For variety, alternate each leg for a total of ten repetitions each leg.

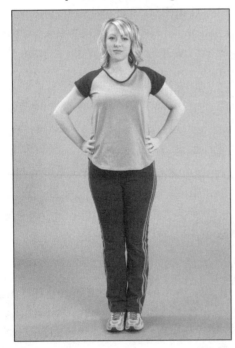

FIGURE 6-1
Starting position for Knee Raises exercise

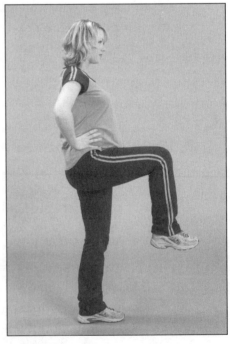

FIGURE 6-2
Raised knee posture

■ Chest Stretch

Stand with your feet together or apart, pelvis tucked in, and abdominals held tightly. Spread your arms to each side, at shoulder level (see **FIGURE 6-3**). Slowly curl your back forward, while bringing your arms forward as well. Allow your head to go forward slowly with this motion but try to keep the tension from your neck (see **FIGURE 6-4**). As you return to a standing pose, spread your arms back to your side and feel the stretch in your chest. To ensure you feel this stretch, pull your shoulder blades together behind your back. Repeat this ten times.

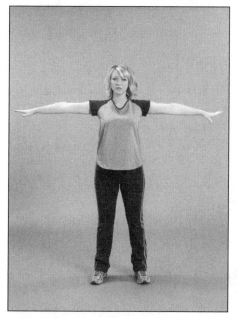

FIGURE 6-3
Starting position for Chest Stretch

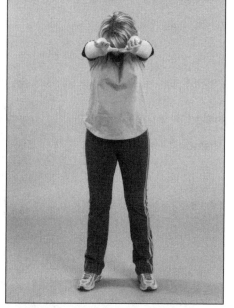

FIGURE 6-4
Hold this position for three to ten seconds. Enjoy the stretch of the upper back and feel the tension draining.

■ Upward Stretch

Stand with your feet about hip-distance apart, with your left hand on your left hip. Reach your opposite arm slowly over your head. To prevent balance problems, try to keep your arm slightly forward of your body. If you still have trouble with balance, step forward slightly with your right foot. Do up to ten repetitions on each side.

■ Side Stretch

With your feet hip-width apart, let your arms hang by your sides. Hold your head up and imagine your spine lengthening. Slowly bend from your waist to the left side of your body. You can hold your right arm slightly away from your body, or you can slide that arm down your leg (see **FIGURE 6-5**). Your left arm can be held away from your body to help you balance if you need it. This will help prevent you from leaning back, which can cause backache as your abdomen grows. Slowly, return to a standing position. Do one on each side (alternating) for a total of twenty repetitions.

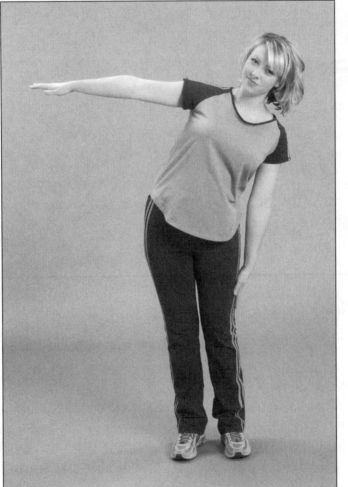

FIGURE 6-5
Side Stretch

■ Upper Back Stretch

Sit on the birth ball with your feet facing forward in front of you. Lift your arms above your head, palms facing forward. Extend your upper back, one vertebra at a time (see **FIGURE 6-6**). As you feel your spine lengthen, you will be stretching your upper back. Now relax one arm to the side, and do each arm at a time. Repeat ten times on each side and finish with both arms stretching again. Have your feet wide enough apart to accommodate your expanding abdomen.

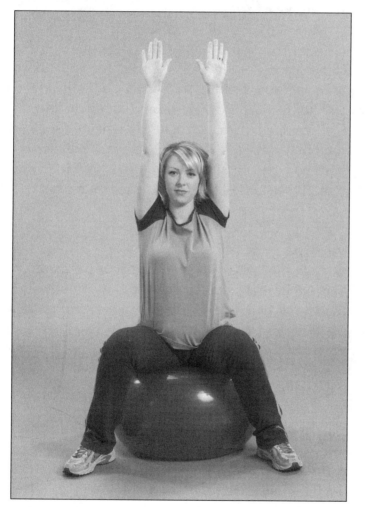

FIGURE 6-6
Upper Back Stretch

Standing Exercises

■ Posture Retraining

Place your back against the wall; slowly walk your feet forward until they are 6 to 8 inches in front of you. Press your glutes, shoulder blades, and the back of your head into the wall (see **FIGURE 5-3**, p. 59). Slowly raise your arms at a 90-degree angle, bent elbow to the wall, and press them to the wall as well. Slowly raise your arms, keeping them on the wall, above your head (see **FIGURE 5-4**, p. 59).

■ Lunge

Stand up without the support of the wall. Maintain the proper posture while stepping back with your left leg. Your upper body should remain facing forward and not moving. Be sure to keep your right knee above your right ankle, as leaning or twisting could cause injury (see **FIGURE 5-5**, p. 60). Lower your body until your right thigh is nearly parallel to the floor. Raise up your body by pressing into your right foot (see **FIGURE 5-6**, p. 60). Do about ten repetitions of this exercise and then repeat on the opposite side.

■ Heel Extensions

Standing with your feet shoulder-width apart and your hands on your hips, bend your right knee and straighten that leg out to the front, with your left knee soft. Touch your right heel to the floor and return to standing. As you move your feet, raise your arms over your head, returning them to your hips as you bring your feet back to the beginning pose. Repeat this exercise ten times on each side. If you need a lower intensity, keep your hands on your hips rather than raising them over your head.

Sitting and Lying Exercises

■ Bridge on Ball

While sitting on a birth ball, (see **FIGURE 6-7**) slowly walk your feet in front of you until the ball is between your shoulder blades (see **FIGURE 6-8**). Keep your ankles in line with your knees and be careful not to extend your knees farther than your toes. Keep your feet as wide apart as needed to maintain your balance. When you achieve this balance, squeeze your abdominal muscles, gluteal muscles, and hamstrings as you breathe, and hold the position for three to five breaths. Lower your hips after you've achieved that number of breaths, then assume the position again. Repeat it ten times.

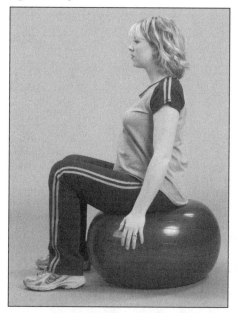

◀ **FIGURE 6-7**
Sitting on a birth ball

FIGURE 6-8 ▼
This helps improve balance and stability by building your abdominal muscles and back.

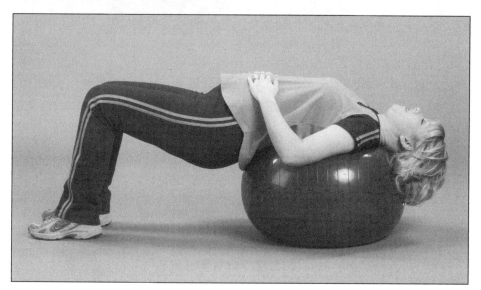

Seated Row

Sitting on the floor with a flex band wrapped around your feet at the middle of the band, hold one end of the band in each hand (see **FIGURE 6-9**). Your palms should be facing the floor. Pull the bands to your chest. Slowly release the tension in the band, returning to the original pose. Repeat this rowing motion ten times.

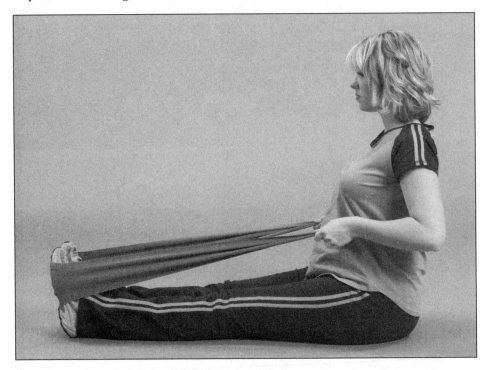

FIGURE 6-9
Hold this position for three to ten seconds.

Cat Balance

While kneeling on the floor, pull in your abdominal muscles and breathe naturally. As you exhale, extend your right leg and left arm. Think about extending each limb as far as you comfortably can. Hold this pose for three to five breaths. Repeat ten times on each side.

■ The Figure Eight

Sitting upright on your birth ball, place your hands on your hips. Imagine what a figure eight looks like. Begin your figure eight by leading with the left hip, going to the right, and backward diagonally, still with your left hip, then switch to lead with your right hip up and back until your figure eight is completed. You should be able to do this more fluidly as you practice. This exercise feels great and helps you get those kinks out of your sides.

■ Pelvic Rock/Pelvic Tilt

This is the perfect exercise for backaches in pregnancy. It will not only help prevent them, but will cure them as well. Assume an all-fours position, on your hands and knees. Think of holding your back in its natural alignment (see **FIGURE 5-7**, p. 61). Then tuck only your pelvis in, bringing your pubic bone toward your neck. Be sure to move only your pelvis (see **FIGURE 5-8**, p. 61). If it helps, have someone hold your pelvis so that you can learn to isolate this area. Later, this exercise can be done in different positions. You need to do two sets of twenty repetitions of the pelvic tilts.

For an added bonus, do another set of twenty repetitions just before bed to help you sleep. For variety, do this exercise while sitting on a birth ball.

■ Squat

This can help strengthen the muscles of your thighs to allow for an easier time at birth if you choose to give birth in this position. Start by using a chair or a partner and stand facing him or her with your feet shoulder-width apart. Slowly lower your body, as he lowers his. Go down as far as you can, while keeping your heels on the floor (see **FIGURE 5-9**, p. 62). You will probably require some practice doing this exercise until you can do it alone and go down into a near sitting position. Do ten squats, holding each one five to ten seconds. Avoid bouncing in between squats.

■ Neck Roll-ups

Lie on the floor on your back as flat as you can. Tilt your pelvis up, so that your spine is flat on the floor. Slowly begin to curl your body up from the chin to the neck, bringing your head with your chin. Pull up until your shoulder blades are off the floor (see **FIGURE 5-10**, p. 62). Hold this pose for five to ten seconds. Repeat ten times.

■ Hip Abduction Lying

Lie on your back with your knees bent, feet flat on the floor and your shoulders and hips placed firmly on the floor. Place your right ankle on your left knee. Bring your left knee toward your chest by grabbing your left thigh with your left hand (see **FIGURE 5-11**, p. 63). Hold this for about five seconds. Repeat on the opposite side.

■ Cat Pose

Get on your hands and knees on the floor with your spine straight, not bowed. As you exhale, lift your right arm and left leg, extending each, as you think about contracting the muscles in the raised arm and in your glutes (see **FIGURE 5-13**, p. 64). Hold this pose for up to five seconds, releasing it on an exhale breath. Return to the starting position and repeat using your opposite limbs.

Cool-down

Remember, the goal is to bring your body down slowly from its excited exercise state. Ending your cool-down with mental relaxation is important as well. Consider doing more pelvic tilts, as well as going through the entire stretching motions. To this add:

■ Side Lying Stretches

Lying on your right side, stretch your right arm over your body as if reaching for something above your head. Focus on extending the arm as well at the leg and body (see **FIGURE 5-14**, p. 65). This should feel like a good tension release. Hold this pose for about ten seconds. Repeat on the left side.

Relaxation Techniques

Relaxation is still a very important part of your pregnancy workout. If you've become attached to one particular position for exercise, work very hard on trying other positions. You can even learn to do mental and emotional relaxation while sitting at your desk or on a birth ball.

Involve Your Partner

See if you can get your partner to help you do your relaxation exercises. This will help you as you prepare to work together during the labor and birth of your baby. Try to do this several times a week, and not always at bedtime.

If you can have your partner help you with the relaxation, also try to "write" a scenario together for you to be led through during a relaxation session. By doing this together, you can find one that works well for both of you. This way, no one winds up rolling in laughter on the floor during labor.

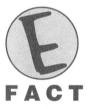

FACT

If you are having a hard time trying to find experiences to talk about during relaxation practices, do not worry. You can start by using simple affirmations or even reading scripts from books and childbirth class. This is perfectly acceptable.

One technique you can do is to have your partner remind you of a favorite vacation, romantic dinner, or any other nice time you've had together. Remember to hit all of your senses when you write this scene. It should include how you felt physically, what you were wearing, what sounds you heard, smells that were present . . . basically anything you can remember. This works better if it's something that you've actually lived through.

Another idea is to have your partner tell you about the birth of your baby. I call this the ideal birth exercise. While this exercise is not one that you've actually lived through, the repetition of this scene can help you refine your ideal birth and become more accepting of alternatives. This also plays to the power of positive thinking. By reminding yourself of a healthy, positive experience, you can actually help make that a reality and feel more comfortable with the experience to come. Ⓔ

Chapter 7

Your Third Trimester

As you prepare for the final months of pregnancy and the beginning of your new life with the baby, your mind and body become preoccupied. This period of time is one when exercise will help you focus on the tasks at hand as well as on keeping your body tuned for the labor day. If you find yourself slowing down, don't worry; it's normal. You'll begin to conserve your energies for your upcoming changes.

Exercise Barriers in the Third Trimester

The third trimester is radically different from the second. Many women find that overnight they feel larger and more weighed down by pregnancy complaints. The good news is that this period of time is when your baby is gaining weight, and developing brown fat to help them regulate their body temperature. Their lungs are also maturing rapidly.

All of these changes are great signs that pregnancy is progressing. Your uterus will rapidly expand to accommodate your growing baby. Your baby will gain about 5 pounds during this trimester. This means that you need to remain ever vigilant about your nutrition, particularly the protein, as it's the building block of every cell. Hydration will also help prevent preterm labor contractions.

As you would expect with all of these changes going on inside the uterus, your body must adapt. Exercise will help you alleviate and prevent many of the common complaints of late pregnancy. However, there are some barriers to fitness that are unique to this stage of pregnancy.

Fatigue and Insomnia

As you get closer to your due date, you may find that fatigue and insomnia once again begin to plague you. These complaints are very common for pregnant women. However, these problems can also be caused by physical or emotional reasons.

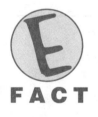

FACT

Trying to determine if you're staying awake at night because of your mind racing or physical issues can be a tough call. But the benefits to you and your baby make the question worth asking. It can also help you solve the problems that are preventing you from getting a good night's rest.

When timed appropriately, physical activity will help increase your ability to sleep. So if your problem is really a physical one, doing exercises or your fitness routine, however modified, should be done prior to the evening hours. Exercising just before bed can make sleep nearly impossible. The physical exercises can also help you address problem areas. For example, good stretches can help you alleviate and prevent backaches.

If you determine that the cause of your wakefulness is more mental and emotional, the relaxation exercises you can do will often help you learn to put these thoughts out of your mind. Training your mind to focus on certain topics will also be beneficial in labor. The ability to focus internally and deal with what the need is at hand is very useful. That's not to say you shouldn't address issues and concerns, just don't do it at bedtime.

While medications may not be useful in trying to help you turn in at night, there are other things to try. Old remedies like a warm bath (but not too warm) and a good book really can help. Sometimes practicing your labor relaxation just before bed can make it easier to fall asleep. Even the proverbial glass of milk can be helpful.

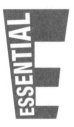

Dreams as a part of pregnancy are often hard to shake. While some may be funny, others may be your way of expressing your worst fears about parenting. Either way, keeping a dream journal next to your bed to write down your dreams can help you deal with them when you're awake.

Return of Nausea

Feeling nauseated is enough to make anyone want to lie in bed all day. Unfortunately for some women, the return of nausea and vomiting in the third trimester is a reality. Be prepared to deal with it should it rear its ugly head again.

The cause of the nausea and vomiting is thought to be partially hormonal, as it was in your first trimester. However, the third trimester brings about a new issue—the baby. Sometimes the pressure of the baby's growing body and the expanding uterus on your other organs is enough to cause your stomach to be upset.

You might find that eating smaller meals will help you avoid some of these issues. You also need to try eating more frequently to make up for the smaller meals. This ensures that you and the baby are still getting adequate nutrition.

Heartburn

You might also find that nausea and vomiting are connected with heartburn. Heartburn is what you call it when you experience a burning sensation in your esophagus. It is caused from the relaxation of the sphincter muscle that guards the stomach. The relaxation is caused by the hormones of pregnancy.

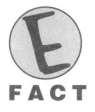

FACT

Papaya enzymes can help alleviate pain and irritation from heartburn. You can try eating papaya fruit, drinking papaya juice, or even taking papaya tablets. These enzymes help with digestion.

When you experience this relaxation of the sphincter muscle, stomach acids are able to leak out of the stomach and into the esophagus. This is what causes the irritation. At the end of your pregnancy, the growing uterus also places a lot of pressure on your organs. This can also encourage the escape of stomach acids into the esophagus. The good news is that there are many things you can do to help with the pain and even elimination of heartburn:

- Eat smaller meals.
- Remain upright after you eat.
- Avoid greasy or spicy foods.
- Avoid foods that seem to bring on heartburn.
- Eat more frequently throughout the day and evening.
- Try a glass of milk or a teaspoon of honey to help alleviate pain.

Blood Pressure

Blood pressure issues in pregnancy usually cause a big debate. Although true blood pressure problems are contraindications to working out during your pregnancy, many of the issues raised in pregnancy are merely unknowns. The biggest debate is what constitutes a blood pressure problem.

Let me start by saying that true blood pressure problems are very serious and need to be addressed immediately. High blood pressure can reduce blood flow to the placenta and the baby, which can lead to Fetal Growth Restriction (FGR). It can also cause the placenta to age prematurely. In very severe cases, the mom can have a stroke, or the placenta can pull away from the wall of the uterus before it is supposed to do so. This is called *placental abruption*.

These problems are all potentially life-threatening to you and your baby, and must be addressed quickly and efficiently by your medical team. If you believe you're having a problem, do not hesitate to call your doctor or midwife immediately.

ALERT!

White coat hypertension is when your blood pressure goes up when you see your doctor or midwife. It sounds unbelievable, but it does occur and it can lead to added interventions, even when there really isn't a blood pressure issue. Ask to use a twenty-four-hour monitor to assess your true blood pressure readings throughout the day to determine if you have white coat hypertension or the real variety.

Most women do not experience these types of problems. Rather, they experience a slow, upward progression of their blood pressure readings. Although your blood pressure numbers might be great for someone else, they could be high readings for you. That is why it is so important to always compare blood pressures to your earlier prenatal visits. The most important will be the rate of rise from the middle trimester.

Special Considerations

The final stretch of the pregnancy journey has finally begun. As you've learned to adapt to the physical and mental changes throughout pregnancy, the third trimester is no different. There are also specific things going on this trimester that you need to be aware of as you work out.

Clumsiness and Lack of Motivation

If you thought you were clumsy last trimester, just wait! Your bulging belly is beautiful, but it can also cause you to take unnecessary spills if you're not careful. Wear sensible shoes, and watch for hazards, such as wet floors.

The third trimester might also be one when you have days of not wanting to do much of anything. Or you might want to divert your energies into preparing your baby's space in your home. Either way, it's okay to take days off. Remember that motivation will come and go, particularly in this third trimester. Your mind will wander and you'll have other things to focus on. Give yourself the space to take time off.

ESSENTIAL

If you feel like taking time off but really don't want to do that in the same breath, consider modifying your workout. Perhaps you can do a warmup and cool-down, rather than the entire workout. Maybe it's time for a change in your workout. Rather than doing your aerobics today, go for a swim instead.

Feeling Overwhelmed

Feeling overwhelmed can also play a big part in lack of motivation. You've got the pregnancy and impending birth on your mind. Perhaps you're concerned about your job, or maybe you've even taken other big plunges, like a new home or other investments. These all weigh heavily when trying to focus on anything. A change in pace or activity can help. Remember, however, that exercise can help you experience less insomnia, and fewer side effects from your pregnancy.

Learning to Slow Down

As your pregnancy draws near the end, you are probably learning that taking things a bit more easily is wise. Sometimes your body forces you to take it easy. Other times it's the natural progression of the cycle of pregnancy.

No matter why you decide to slow down or when, in the third trimester, it's important to recognize this as a good thing. Easing up on your fitness routines gives your body a chance to finish the pregnancy and prepare for labor, birth, and postpartum.

Exercises for the Third Trimester

The precautions for the third trimester include watching for signs of preterm labor, dehydration, safety issues, and symptoms of maternal supine hypotension syndrome. If you have any complications from these or other things that arise in your workout, stop exercising immediately. Call your doctor or midwife to discuss possible modifications.

Your prenatal appointments will be much more frequent at this point in your pregnancy. Be sure to ask your practitioner about exercise every visit to ensure you're both on the same page. This will also help both of you stay informed about your abilities and exercises.

There are no specific recommendations to stop exercising prior to labor. Many women go through pregnancy and exercise until the day of labor. Other moms might feel tired and worn-out, decreasing their workouts in intensity and frequency as they go. Either way is fine as long as it is what is right for you and your baby.

Warmups and Cool-downs

Your warmup during the third trimester really sets the tone for your whole workout. There will be days that you do the warmup and decide that's enough. The important thing to remember is to listen to your body. Again the warmup helps protect you from injury, so don't skip it in the interest of saving time or energy.

Your cool-down won't change, except perhaps to make it longer. Your body is slower to make transitions at this stage of pregnancy. Be sure to always include some mental relaxation as a way to stay focused on the mind-body connection.

Mind-Body Connection

The mind-body connection is something you've really been working on throughout your pregnancy. As you've practiced your relaxation and listened to your body, you've probably noticed a greater connection between the way your mind and body work together. The healthier you feel physically, the easier it is to feel better mentally.

ESSENTIAL

The confidence you've gained from your fitness routines and the strength in your body will give you strength and faith in the same body for labor, birth, and parenting. Remember to draw on these strengths as you go forward.

Preparing for Labor

Your strong mind and body, which you've spent the last nine months or more preparing for this grand adventure, will not fail you. Remember to listen to the signals as you have done throughout your pregnancy fitness sessions. Follow your body's lead and be prepared to go with the flow. Mind and body, and flexibility and knowledge will go a long way toward making your labor and birth experience a great one to remember for the rest of your life.

Relaxation

Mental imagery is one form of relaxation that can be effectively used in labor. As with all of the relaxation techniques you learn, practice makes perfect. The mental imagery requires a bit more imagination or recollection on your part, however.

Using a dream location or a previous vacation spot are frequent scenarios couples choose to use in doing mental imagery. While this works for many people, don't be concerned if going to the beach or into the forest doesn't work for you. There isn't a right or wrong answer for what mental images you use.

Another popular technique for mental imagery is to think of what your body is doing during labor. This works really well if you are someone who needs to focus on the process and be aware of what is going on inside your body. Examples to think about might be an image of a cervix opening up or of your baby moving down into the pelvis.

Problem Spots

Don't be concerned if you've tried a variety of relaxations and not all of them work. Remember, we are each different individuals who respond differently to different situations. If you're particularly good at one, keep that one ever present. If there are some that don't work or sound funny, try them once or twice in case they do work in labor. Otherwise, you can skip those once you're familiar with them.

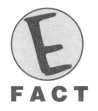

FACT

According to a long-term study of women's memories of giving birth to their children, childbirth educator Penny Simkin found that even after twenty-five years, the memories of what was said or done on this day stuck with the women as if it were only yesterday. This will be an important day in your life.

Sample Exercise Program

The exercises listed here are generally fine for the third trimester of pregnancy. Remember to modify any exercises as you see fit, and skip those that cause pain. Show these exercises to your doctor or midwife if you have any questions about the exercises themselves or your ability to participate in the exercises.

Warmup

Try all of these exercises or a combination of them for your warmup.

■ Hip Stretches

Keeping a chair to your right side for balance, stand with your feet shoulder-width apart (see **FIGURE 7-1**). Begin by resting your right hand on the chair and your left hand on your hip. Take a step backward with your left leg. Your weight should be distributed evenly between your feet. Lift the heel of your left foot. Slightly bend both of your knees and do an exaggerated pelvic tilt while holding on to the chair (see **FIGURE 7-2**). Repeat this exercise five times on each side.

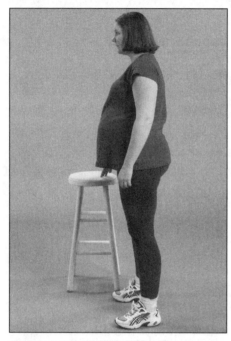

FIGURE 7-1
Hip Stretches

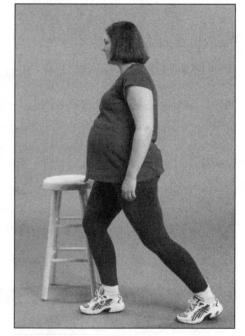

FIGURE 7-2
This stretch will also help with restless legs and aches.

■ Neck Stretch

Stand with your feet shoulder-width apart. Let your shoulders be held up and back. The crown of your head should be pulling upward. Slowly let your chin drop to your chest and hold it there for five to ten seconds. Return your head to the neutral position. Slowly let your left ear rest on your left shoulder, again holding it for five to ten seconds. Repeat this on your right side. It is okay if you can't hold your head all the way down. Move until you feel the stretch, but without pain. Do this series three to five times.

Middle Chest Stretch

With your feet about shoulder-width apart, place your hands on your lower back, just above your buttocks. Slowly begin to stretch backward as you try to pull your shoulder blades and elbows together. Hold this pose for about five to ten seconds. Repeat the stretch up to ten times. Be sure to keep your chin level and your head facing forward. Always tuck in your abdominal muscles.

Wrist/Ankle Rotations

While holding your body in its correct posture, extend your arms in front of you. They should be at your chest level, just below your shoulder. Rotate your wrists forward and backward, about ten small circles each direction. This can be particularly good to try before bed. If you find yourself suffering from repetitive motion syndrome (RSS) or carpal tunnel syndrome (CTS), try these stretches before beginning your work day and every few hours to relieve pain. Repeat the same exercise with your ankles.

Knee Raises

Stand with a chair to one side of your body and keep your feet shoulder-width apart, placing the hand closest to the chair on its back. The other hand should be on your hip. While maintaining your proper posture, lift the knee farthest from the chair slightly outward until it is at about a 90-degree angle (see **FIGURE 6-2**, p. 78). Slowly lower your leg. Repeat this exercise for a total of ten repetitions and then switch knees for another ten repetitions.

Marching

Stand with your feet slightly apart and your arms loosely at your side. Begin by marching, or exaggerated walking, by bringing your knees up one at a time and returning it to the floor, alternating feet. You should take care not to stomp your feet down and not to raise your knees above a comfortable height.

Calf Stretch

With your hands on your hips and your feet shoulder-width apart, point your toes forward (see **FIGURE 7-3**). Step backward with your right foot. The step length should be comfortable and yet a stretch. Ensuring your posture is aligned properly, lean forward, making sure your knee does not extend over your foot (see **FIGURE 7-4**). This stretch will be felt in the calf of your rear leg. Do ten of these repetitions and then repeat on the opposite side. If you find yourself in need of some stability while you do this exercise, use a chair placed to one side of your body to hang on to, or even use a wall in front of you.

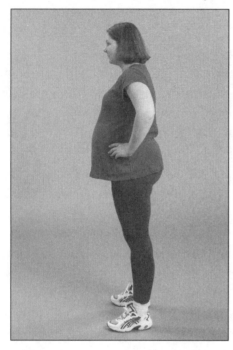

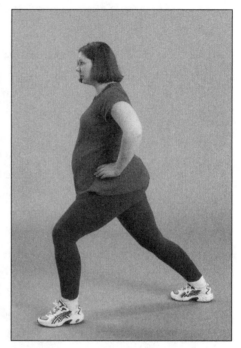

FIGURE 7-3
Calf Stretches

FIGURE 7-4
Done before bed, this stretch can prevent nighttime charley horses.

■ Side Stretch

Sit on the birth ball with your feet facing forward in front of you. Extend your right arm over your head, with your palm facing your left side. Your left hand should be on the side of the ball. Slowly lean toward your left side, extending your arm and letting the ball move slightly as you lean (see **FIGURE 8-3**, p. 116). When you've reached your maximum stretch, hold this pose for five seconds and then return to your upright position. Do a total of five repetitions of this exercise. Repeat the same movement with the opposite side.

Standing Exercises

■ Standing Hip Abduction

This exercise should start with a wall, until you learn your body's balance. Make sure the wall is on your right side, and place your hand palm-side down on the wall for support. Shift your weight to the right leg, lifting your left leg to the side about 10 to 12 inches (see **FIGURE 7-5**). This is not a large movement. Do ten repetitions and repeat on the opposite side.

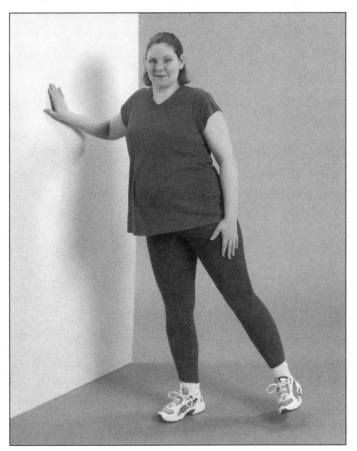

FIGURE 7-5
Standing Hip Abduction

■ Wall Squat

Standing up straight with your back facing a wall, place the birth ball between you and the wall around the center of your back and press it into the wall using your back. Slowly walk your feet forward, leaning back into the ball for support (see **FIGURE 7-6**). As you walk forward, the ball will roll up to the center of your back, between your shoulder blades. This allows you to do a squat without having to worry about being steady or having a partner (see **FIGURE 7-7**). When you are down as far as you can go, hold the pose for up to ten seconds, then slowly walk your feet back to their starting position allowing the ball to roll back to the center of your lower back.

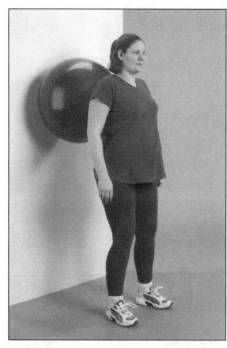

FIGURE 7-6
Wall Squat

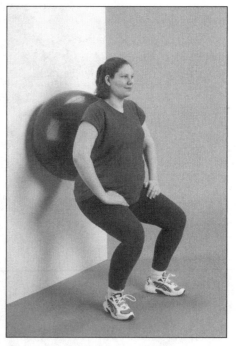

FIGURE 7-7
This squat is great for when your belly is too big to comfortably squat traditionally, or even for beginners.

■ Knee Raises

Stand with your feet shoulder-width apart. Watch your posture and pull your abdominals inward. Lift your left knee slightly outward to avoid your belly, tap your knee with your right hand. Alternate knee raises until you've done ten repetitions on each side.

■ Side Taps

Standing with your feet together and your hands to your side (see **FIGURE 7-8**), bend your left knee and raise the opposite leg to the side. Touch your toes to the floor (see **FIGURE 7-9**). Return to starting pose. Repeat this exercise five to ten times on each side, depending on your energy or fitness level. Use your arms as needed for balance.

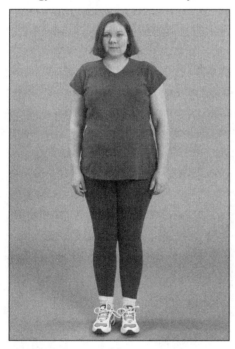

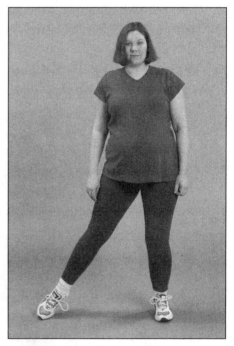

FIGURE 7-8
Side Taps

FIGURE 7-9
This is a great way to stretch and strengthen your outer thighs.

Sitting and Lying Exercises

■ Kegels on Ball

While sitting on a birth ball and maintaining your posture, be sure your abdominal muscles are pulled in. Focus on your breathing as you practice Kegeling while on the ball. Do fifteen to twenty repetitions of whatever variety of Kegels you have worked up to at this point in your pregnancy.

■ Double Arm Lifts

Stand in the middle of your flex band. Hold one end of the band in each hand, while your arms hang by your sides. Relax and bend your knees slightly, while maintaining your spine in an upright position. Slowly, and together, raise both hands to your sides, palms upward, until you reach shoulder level. Do this exercise for ten repetitions.

■ Kneeling Abdominal Curl

Kneeling on the floor with your hands forward, palms down, tilt your pelvis in, pulling your belly toward the center of your body (see **FIGURE 7-10**). Hold this pose for a count of ten. Repeat ten times. You can also do this by leaning across a chair to support your upper body.

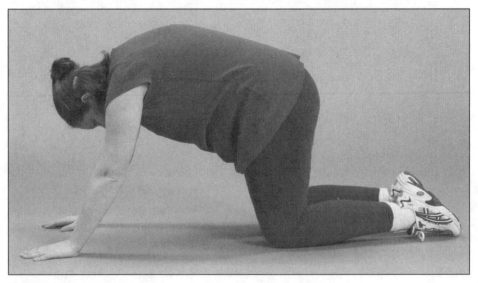

FIGURE 7-10
Kneeling Abdominal Curl

■ Step Touch

Stand with your feet together and your arms at your side. In the next movement, step to your side with your right foot as both of your arms go to shoulder height. This should be a smooth movement to avoid problems with injury. Step to the left and move your arms again to your shoulders. Do twenty alternating steps, which will give you ten repetitions on each side. To add intensity, consider adding arm movements to the step touch beyond just lifting to shoulder height. You can add a biceps curl, and extension forward with your arms and hands or any other variation that works for you. Remember that adding arm movements increases intensity.

■ Abdominal Tightening

Sitting on a birth ball, place your hands on your abdomen. Tilt your pelvis, and as you inhale, pull your abdominal muscles inward. Feel your abdomen muscles move as your hands rest on them. Hold the pose for five seconds, while breathing. Repeat this exercise ten times.

■ Hip Abduction Lying

Lie on your back with your knees bent, feet flat on the floor and your shoulders and hips firmly on the floor. Place your right ankle on your left knee. Bring your left knee toward your chest by grabbing your left thigh with your left hand (see **FIGURE 5-11**, p. 63). Hold this for about five seconds. Repeat on the opposite side.

■ Child's Pose

Kneel on the floor, separating your knees slightly, or as much as is needed to have your belly fall comfortably between your knees. Put your big toes together and sit back with your buttocks on the heels of your feet. Stretch your arms over your head, and stop at a resting place on your forearms (see **FIGURE 5-12**, p. 63). Hold this pose for five seconds, releasing a bit more with each breath. If this reach is not enough of a stretch for you, lie your arms all the way down on the ground.

Cool-down

Many people simply do the their warm-up for their cool-down. However, you can add more exercises to this section because your body is already stretched and warmed up. Remember, the goal is to bring your body down slowly from its excited exercise state. Ending your cool-down with mental relaxation is important as well. Consider doing more pelvic tilts, as well as going through the entire stretching motions. To this add:

■ Seated Pectoral Stretch

While tailor sitting on the floor or seated on a birth ball, place your hands on your lower back above your buttocks. Concentrate on pulling your shoulder blades together and continue breathing. Do this exercise ten times.

■ Side Lying Stretches

Lying on your right side, stretch your right arm over your body as if reaching for something above your head. Focus on extending the arm as well at the leg and body (see **FIGURE 5-14**, p. 65). This should feel like a good tension release. Hold this pose for about ten seconds. Repeat on the left side.

■ Full Body Extension

Sitting on a birth ball, extend your arms above your head and lengthen your arms, much like the side lying extension. Hold this pose for ten seconds and repeat. You can then choose a position for relaxation.

Relaxation

To begin your relaxation session, choose a position that is good for you. Perhaps you will use the side lying position, or situate yourself propped up on pillows on the floor or your bed. No matter what position you choose, be sure to alternate positions so that you can practice in different positions. Include some seated positions, as well as positions that are lying down.

Once you've found the position that you will use for this practice session, walk yourself through a series of relaxing stages. If the tense-release exercise works for you, you can do this exercise. You might also try a counting exercise. As you exhale, say the number ten out loud, softly. When you say the number, release tension that you find in your body. Inhale normally. As you exhale again, say nine, again releasing tension. Do this until you've finished with number one. At the end of this period, you should be significantly more relaxed than when you started.

Now that your body is relaxed, focus on a blank screen in your mind, like a movie or television screen. Think of your favorite color. What images pop into your mind? For example, if red is your favorite color, what image pops up? An apple? A schoolhouse? Perhaps a sports car? What feelings and sensations do you have as you think about this object? Do you feel full and warm? Any positive feelings are good. If so, this color works for you. If you have negative feelings, avoid this color or image.

The point of this exercise is to help you relax and be able to conjure up positive images. Using this exercise can help you reframe your day, or even allay your fears during times of stress or trouble. You can do this anywhere and at any time.

Chapter 8

Tools for Toning

Keeping your body toned in pregnancy is not as difficult as it sounds. There are plenty of tools available to help you not only retain muscle tone, but gain strength as well. Finding the right tool for your body and using it correctly are the keys to maintaining a healthy body in pregnancy.

Using Exercise Tools

Exercise is mostly about how you use your body to obtain a level of fitness to keep you healthy and feeling good. Many people do this without the use of any special equipment. However, using tools to aid in your workout can keep the workout fresh and helps prevent you from growing bored with the same routine. Adding variety can also help ensure a balanced workout for your entire body.

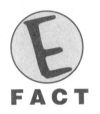

FACT

Using different tools in your workout will help you add variety to keep your workouts interesting. They can also add different exercises and resistance training that you may not be able to get elsewhere during your pregnancy. When used properly, they are a safe and effective set of training tools in pregnancy.

Weights

Weights have long been used to aid in exercise programs. Many women are accustomed to working out with weights prior to pregnancy. Until recently, it was believed that weight training didn't belong in a prenatal exercise program. Today, we understand that there can be a benefit to weight training in pregnancy with a few simple precautions.

Free Weights

Free weights are weights you can actually pick up and use while exercising. You may think of these as barbells or hand weights, but it can also be something as simple as ankle and wrist weights, which can be used in exercises for the arms and legs to increase resistance and improve muscle tone.

Machines

Machines can also be used in pregnancy, but you need to be well trained and you must follow the appropriate instructions for each one. Some machines will not be appropriate for every stage of pregnancy, particularly those that require lying on your stomach. Be sure to talk to the fitness instructor as well as your physician about the use of weight machines in pregnancy.

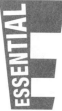

Using weights in pregnancy is fine, though you should ease up on the amounts of weights you lift as you get further along. To prevent injury, you might switch to using machines only in your third trimester when your balance is likely to be at its worst.

Since weightlifting is so popular, Chapter 12 is devoted to additional information on weightlifting and pregnancy.

Flex Bands

Flex bands are used to help increase flexibility and can be used to create resistance in your exercise programs. They are lightweight, inexpensive, and easy to find. This makes them easier to use during pregnancy for many women. They are also great to use when trying to maintain your fitness while on the road, whether traveling for work or pleasure.

Buying Your Flex Bands

The bands can be purchased at stores that specialize in fitness or sporting goods, or they can be ordered through many catalogues. They do come in a variety of shapes, sizes, and resistance levels. The bands are very economical, usually costing just a few dollars each.

If you can, purchase at least two different resistance levels, for example, light and medium. If offered different lengths, look for something in the 4-foot range. This gives you more exercise options, particularly when working around your increasing abdomen.

How to Use Them

To care for your bands, be sure to store them away from direct light, whether it be sunlight or room light. Extremes in light and temperature can be damaging to the elastic materials. You can wash them by wetting them and then hanging them up to dry without the use of light or heat. Be sure to inspect your bands often for signs of tears, holes, weakened areas, and splits. The bands will eventually wear out and need to be replaced. Do replace your bands if you find any of these problems. Using a band that is defective can injure you.

Exercises with the Flex Bands

Exercising with the flex bands can be a lot of fun. If you keep in mind the rules of using the flex bands, you should have a great tool to add to your workout. They are also simple enough that you can take them on trips, use them in the office, or just about anywhere you might be located.

■ Single Arm Lifts

Stand with one foot slightly forward, and your feet about shoulder-width apart. Stand on your flex band with your right foot, while grasping the other end of the band with your right hand (see **FIGURE 8-1**). With your palm

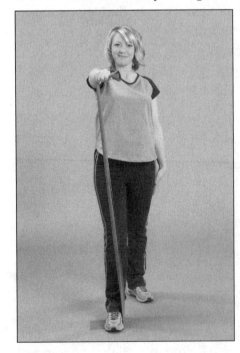

FIGURE 8-1
Single Arm Lifts

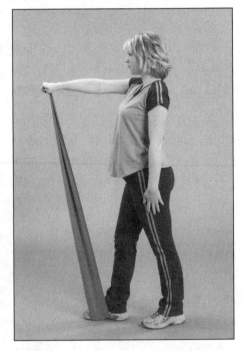

FIGURE 8-2
Remember to pull the band slowly to maximize muscle use and prevent injury.

down, slowly raise the right arm to shoulder level (see **FIGURE 8-2**). Hold this pose for up to five seconds and then slowly lower the right arm. Repeat this motion ten times. Then switch to the left arm.

■ Double Arm Lifts

This exercise is similar to the single arm lift, but with emphasis on both arms. To begin this exercise, stand in the middle of your flex band. Hold one end of the band in each hand, while your arms hang by your sides. Relax and bend your knees slightly, while maintaining your spine in an upright position. Slowly, and together, raise both hands to your sides, palms upward, until you reach shoulder level. Be careful to use only your arms and not your shoulders in this exercise. The goal is to strengthen your arms to help you gain strength for tasks such as lifting your new baby. Do this exercise for ten repetitions.

■ Side Arm Stretches

Stand with your feet shoulder-width apart. Take the flex band in both hands, with your palms facing upward. Your arms and elbows should be tucked into your sides. Hold the left hand steady as you move the right forearm and hand slowly away from your body. Follow your natural range of motion here, and don't overdo it. When you reach your limit, slowly bring your right hand back to its starting position. Repeat this exercise ten times. Switch to your left hand, moving it while your right hand remains steady.

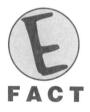

FACT

You can combine many of the flex band exercises and others to be used with the birth ball. Anything that can be done while standing can usually be done sitting on the birth ball for exercise. This takes some of the pressure off if you're looking for a less intense workout, particularly as your pregnancy advances. Remember, never hesitate to modify your workout.

The Birth Ball

The birth ball is also known as a physiotherapy ball. While it might look hilarious as an exercise tool, it is very helpful. These physiotherapy or birth balls have long been used in physical therapy for helping gain and maintain strength and flexibility in patients. Now that their popularity is catching on, you can find them in most fitness facilities, not to mention birthing rooms!

These birth balls are used as an integral part of exercise programs all over the world. There are even classes designed solely using the balls. They can be used for posture, balance, tone, and other reasons to help make your exercise safe and fun.

Birth Ball Benefits

Using a ball in your everyday life can actually help alleviate pregnancy complaints. Something as simple as replacing your office chair with a birth ball can really make a difference in your posture and how you feel. Your posture is improved because you can't really slouch well on a birth ball and maintain your balance, so you are forced to sit upright.

The ball also allows for less pressure on your perineum and sensitive pelvis in general. This can be really important, particularly in the final months of pregnancy when your pelvis hurts from sitting on a hard surface.

During labor and birth, the birth balls are used to help find positions for you to assume that are more comfortable. They also allow your baby to be born more easily. Many hospitals and birth centers now equip their facilities with the balls. If your hospital doesn't have its own, bring one from home!

After you give birth, the ball can once again be used in your exercise routine. However, I've also never met kids who didn't enjoy the ball themselves. Babies can even be rocked on the ball to soothe tummies that are rumbling with gas.

Where to Buy and How to Use It

Buying a birth ball isn't that difficult. There are many places you can order a birth ball from, including fitness facilities or medical supply stores in your area.

You will want to ensure, however, that you choose the ball that is the right size for you. When in doubt, the 65-centimeter round ball is a fairly generic shape and size. Be sure to check the weight limits of the ball. Some may go as high as 1,000 pounds, while others are much lower. Do not choose a ball that will hold below 300 pounds. If you are less than 5 feet, 5 inches tall, you might consider the 55-centimeter ball. Likewise, if you are over 6 feet tall, you will want to choose the 75-centimeter ball.

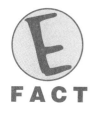

FACT

You can use a standard bike pump with an adaptor to fill your ball, or many balls come with their own pump. To test your ball for under-inflation, sit on it and it should give slightly but not depress too much under your body weight.

Exercises with the Birth Ball

There are many exercises you can do with your birth ball. Here are a few that are good for any point in your pregnancy and recovery. Feel free to add your own to this list and to be creative when using your ball.

■ Upper Back Stretch on the Ball

Sit on the ball with your feet facing forward in front of you. Lift your arms above your head, palms facing forward. Extend your upper back, one vertebra at a time (see **FIGURE 6-6**, p. 81). As you feel your spine lengthen, you will be stretching your upper back. Now, relax one arm to the side, and do each arm singly. Repeat ten times on each side and finish with both arms stretching again.

■ Side Stretch on the Ball

Sit on the ball with your feet facing forward in front of you. Extend your right arm over your head, with your palm facing your left side. Your left hand should be on the side of the ball. Slowly lean toward your left side, extending your arm and letting the ball move slightly as you lean (see **FIGURE 8-3**). When you've reached your maximum stretch (it should stretch but not hurt), hold this pose for five seconds and then return to your upright position. Do a total of five repetitions of this exercise. Repeat the same movement with the opposite side.

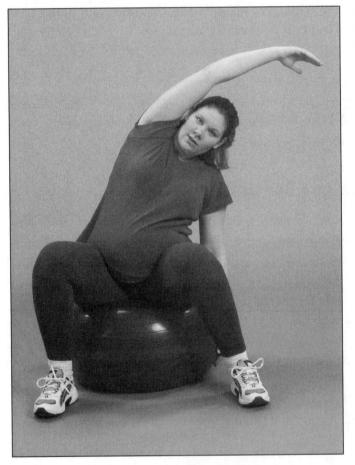

FIGURE 8-3
Side Stretch on the Ball

■ Pelvic Tilts

Sitting upright on the ball, with your arms resting in your lap, simply tilt your pelvis under (see **FIGURE 8-4**). Feel the ball gently sway forward with this movement. You should be able to maintain your balance on the ball while doing this exercise. You can repeat this as often as you like. This will help alleviate and prevent discomfort in your lower back. It can also help rotate your baby if it is in an awkward position prior to or during labor.

You can also do advanced pelvic tilts by sitting upright on the ball and extending your arms to your sides. As you do your pelvic tilts, slowly tuck your pelvis under, and rotate your arms forward in small circles. Feel free to change the size and direction of the circles you make with your arms.

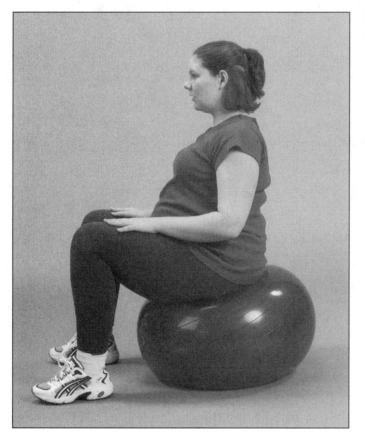

FIGURE 8-4
Pelvic Tilt on the Ball

▧ Hula on the Ball

Sitting upright on the ball, place your hands on your hips and begin to sway your hips from side to side (see **FIGURE 8-5**). How far you go to either side will depend on your comfort and fitness level. This provides a good stretch and gives you a chance to move your body. When you are comfortable with this motion, change your motion to be more of a circular motion (see **FIGURE 8-6**). You can move in either direction, and it's a good idea to actually change directions during your workout. If you're feeling up to it, try yet another variation—the figure eight.

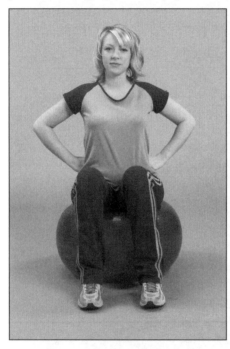

FIGURE 8-5
Hula on the Ball

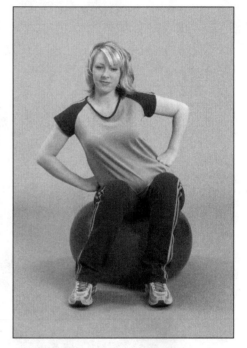

FIGURE 8-6
Doing this exercise slowly helps with the stretch and maintains your balance. Don't go too quickly!

▧ Supported Squat (Wall Squat)

Standing up straight with your back facing a wall, place the birth ball between you and the wall around the center of your back and press it into the wall using your back. Slowly walk your feet forward, leaning back into the ball for support (see **FIGURE 7-6**, p. 102). As you walk forward, the ball will roll up to the center of your back, between your shoulder blades. This allows you to do a squat without having to worry about being steady or having a partner (see **FIGURE 7-7**, p. 102). When you are down as far as you can go, hold the pose for up to ten seconds, then slowly walk your feet back to their starting position allowing the ball to roll back to the center of your lower back.

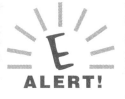

ALERT!

If you ever feel unsteady on the birth ball, be sure you're using it on a dry floor that is not slick. Ensure that you are not wearing socks or other shoes with slippery surfaces, and that the ball is properly inflated. These are all common mistakes made when using a birth ball.

Using the Birth Ball in Labor

Once you've gotten used to using your ball, it will seem only natural to bring it with you to labor. There are many benefits of using the ball in labor:

- Allows movement while supporting you in many positions.
- Comfortable to sit on.
- Encourages your baby into the proper position for birth.
- Encourages upright positioning, allowing maximum blood flow to the placenta and baby.
- Can be used in the shower.
- Can be used during periods of fetal monitoring.
- Can be used in conjunction with light or walking epidurals.
- Can be used in bed.

The flexibility of the birth ball in labor is key to its importance. This doesn't even begin to touch on the physical benefits to you. Using the ball in a variety of positions helps you to relax and go with the flow in labor. It also encourages you to assume comfortable, upright positions, which aid the baby in getting into the proper alignment and allow your body to have maximum blood flow to the placenta.

■ Sitting

Sitting on the ball in labor can help you keep a rhythmic movement going, and allow you to remain upright, even during periods of fetal monitoring.

■ Squatting

This can be done several ways. You can actually squat on the floor while holding on to the ball for support. You can use the ball as a back brace while you squat down using the wall to support the ball. (See Supported Squat, p. 118.) Or, using an egg-shaped ball, be sure to plant your feet slightly wider than usual to achieve the squatting position. These positions help open your pelvis more so that the baby can descend to be born.

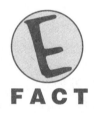

FACT

Squatting in labor is jokingly called the *midwives' forceps*. The reason that this came to be is that by using the squatting position you actually open your pelvic outlet by an additional 10 percent. This added room can help the baby move down toward birth, and often works when other positions have failed.

■ Kneeling

With this position you can place the ball on the floor or the bed for maximum support. Kneel down with the ball in front of you, draping your arms over the ball. You can choose to hold still or you can actually stretch and sway using the ball either during or after contractions.

■ Leaning

Placing the ball on a higher surface, you can stand up and lean over the ball, using it to support your weight. You can also sit on the ball and lean over and hold your partner, or even hold any object. This position takes some of the strain off your back and allows you to stretch out.

Belly Bands

Belly bands or supports are used for a variety of reasons, many of which do not relate directly to exercising. These bands are designed to support your growing abdomen and to allow you more freedom of movement.

They come in a variety of shapes and fashions. Some are simply Velcro enclosures that go around your lower back and secure at your pubic bone. This provides support to your lower back and pubic bone by helping to "hold" your baby up.

There are more complex models that have lower back to pubic bone enclosures, but also encompass the upper body to help alleviate strain and pressure on the shoulders. These also help to remind you of proper posture. Many of these devices can help alleviate some pregnancy related discomforts, though they should not been seen as a replacement for proper exercise and muscle tone. Use them as a support system, not a replacement.

While you do not need a prescription for these items, obtaining one from your doctor or midwife might encourage your insurance company to pay for one. The more complex models can cost about $100. They can be obtained in medical supply stores, some maternity shops, and even online.

If you are expecting a child other than your first, or if you are expecting multiple babies like twins or triplets, these belly bands are great ideas because of the added pressure and distention of your abdominal walls. Talk to your practitioner about using one if you believe it would help you be more comfortable in pregnancy.

Creating Tools from Household Items

While tools have their place in prenatal fitness, they don't have to cost you an arm and a leg. In fact, you can safely make some of these at home without much cost or trouble. Included here a few ideas for some do-it-yourself tools for home exercise.

Weights

Weights are probably some of the simplest things to make. Using an old tube sock and filling it full of coins is a great way to make weights either to carry or even to use as wrist or ankle weights. These can be made as light as you need them to be and you can even add or subtract the weight as you go further in pregnancy.

ALERT!

If you use something, be sure that it is child friendly or that you've put it away where children can't reach it. A sock full of pennies is enticing to a little one, who may then try to eat the coins. The same goes with a bag of sugar or other household item.

Even easier than using pennies in a sock, go to the cupboard. You'd be amazed at how your pantry shelves are stocked with weights. Grab a couple of one-pound (16-ounce) soup cans. One in each hand and you've got one-pound hand weights. Work your way through the cabinets as you progress up to five-pound bags of sugar.

Avoid items that can easily spill or break. For example, a glass container may not be a great weight because if it were to fall, it would shatter. Some people prefer to use specific containers and fill them with items like sand or sugar. You can certainly do this and carefully weigh them out on your bathroom or kitchen scale. This also allows you to choose the shape of the object you will be holding. Ⓔ

Chapter 9

Exercising Your Arms

During pregnancy, you tend to focus on your abdomen, your legs, and maybe your back. However, one of the most often neglected areas is your arms. Learning to exercise this part of your body is simple and not very time-consuming, but the benefits are great!

Why Your Arms Are Important

Most of the exercises you do in pregnancy seem to be geared toward something to help directly with your pregnancy and well-being. However, it is the arms that you really need to focus on, since we use this area of our body all the time but with very little thought. The good news is that very few complications of pregnancy preclude your arm exercises.

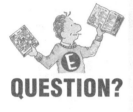

QUESTION?

May I raise my arms above my head while pregnant?
If you are pregnant, you should not lift your arms over your head, so says the common old wives' tale. In doing so, the myth goes, you will cause your baby's umbilical cord to wrap around its neck. This is utter nonsense and should not affect how you work your arms out during pregnancy.

Your arms will be used somewhat in labor, particularly during the pushing phase. You will use them to help pull your legs back or to hold your body up as you push. This can be very tiring if your arms are not used to working out. However, remember that at the end of your hard work, a miracle is placed in these same arms—your baby.

While the work of labor might seem to be enough of a reason to exercise your arms during your pregnancy, there are others. Postpartum is probably the biggest reason to exercise your arms.

During the postpartum phase is when having strong arms is very important. Your arms will be carrying around your new baby and strong arms make that task much easier to bear. Your forearms and wrists will be used repeatedly during the day as you feed, change, and bathe your baby. There is literally no area of the arm that is not used in daily baby care. And that's not even talking about mom care!

Identifying Areas That Need Work

When you think of your arms, you might immediately think of how they look in sleeveless dresses or you might think of strength issues. But truth be told, many of us neglect our arms and pregnant women are no different. Let's look at the different areas of the arm, how they work, and what you can do to make the most out of your arm muscles for fitness and fashion.

Chest Muscles

Women aren't often thought of as having chest muscles. But we do! Ours are simply covered with the breast tissue that helps us nurture our children after birth. The chest muscles are comprised of two muscles: pectoralis major and pectoralis minor.

The pectoralis major is a fan-shaped muscle near the surface that runs horizontally from the middle of your clavicle, or collarbone, to your upper arm. It also encompasses the area from your sternum or breastbone diagonally to the upper arm. This muscle helps you move your arms upward, inward, and across your body.

Working out your chest muscles will not cause you to bulk up. While you will have firmer muscles under your breasts, very few women look like the typical bodybuilder. This will also not significantly change the shape of your breasts, nor interfere with breastfeeding.

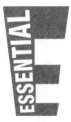

Stretching, particularly before and after feeding your baby, will help release tension in your arms and back. Massage is also a great idea. It's a great way to pamper the new mom, but is also very good for releasing that tension. This can be done by anyone, including a professional masseur or masseuse.

Biceps and Triceps

When you think of arm muscles, the two that are most prominent are the triceps and the biceps, the main muscles in your arms. There are other muscles involved in working out your arms, but focusing on the biceps and triceps will ensure that all these muscles are worked as well.

When working out your arms, it is important to remember to work both the biceps in the front and the triceps in the back equally. If you fail to do this, the muscles are going to develop differently, causing you problems down the road. These muscles work together in an important fashion. Think about bending your arm at the elbow, as your biceps contract to bend the elbow. What happens to the triceps in the rear of your arm? The triceps naturally stretch. This give-and-take is an important balance to visualize and understand.

Your Back and Shoulder Muscles

While you might not think of these muscles as being part of your arms, the chest and back muscles are primary movement makers of your arms. Keeping them strong and healthy will help you with your arm movements and strength. Your back muscles also include the latissimus dorsi, the trapezius muscles, and the rhomboid muscles.

These muscles also assist in holding your body erect. They help provide you support and will help in nursing your baby. Often, a good massage of the upper back before or after a nursing session will be helpful and will feel great.

Forearms

Your forearms are important to pay attention to as well, though we usually forget this portion of the body very quickly. After all, what do the forearms really do for you? They do plenty. The strength of your forearms will determine how strong your grip will be, provides stabilization for your wrists, and provides you with protection from injury of the arm and hand.

As in other chapters, stretching the forearm can be very important, particularly if you use your hands or wrists much in computer work, fine motor skills with your hands, or simply while feeding your baby. The forearms will bear the brunt of all of your arm work.

ALERT!

When working your arms, you need to be sure that you are not extending your arms forcefully or completely. This can actually injure your arm muscles. When doing your exercises, remember to stop just short of a full extension and to use smooth movements to prevent injury.

Hands

Some of the more frequent problems pregnant women experience in their hands are carpal tunnel syndrome and repetitive motion syndrome. Both of these problems are more common in pregnancy. The reason you will see these flare up during pregnancy is because of the added swelling of your tissues.

You may notice a tingling sensation or numbness in your hands and fingers. This can be particularly bad if you work with your hands. If you type a lot at the computer, you are particularly at risk for suffering during pregnancy. If you work at a job where you do the same repetitive motion over and over, then you are also at risk for one of these problems.

However, the good news is that, most of the time, birth will help cure some of your problems with carpal tunnel and repetitive motion syndromes. This is because your body fluid levels will go back to your pre-pregnancy state and relieve some of the added swelling on nerves and the like in your arms and hands. Obviously, if it flares up during pregnancy, you can expect to see it again later in life, during pregnancy or just as you naturally age.

How to Prevent Injuries?

There are a couple of simple solutions and exercises that you can try to prevent carpal tunnel and repetitive motion syndromes from becoming problems. These exercises and strategies also work in helping to alleviate any pain you are already experiencing.

Inspect your workstation by looking around at what is at your desk and how everything is set up. Do you practice good ergonomics? Are you too far away from your keyboard or desk? Ideally, you should be able to keep your arms and elbows relatively close to your body.

Wrist and Hand Protectors

Your wrists should be supported at the keyboard. This can be by using a wrist pad made of several different materials, including gel pads.

This prevents your wrists from being lower than your hands and allows for better circulation and relaxation. You should also have a pad at your mouse.

Wrist splints are also helpful in alleviating pain and complications, although they can be uncomfortable to wear. You can purchase hand splints at most drug stores and physical therapy centers. Many doctors can also prescribe splints that are specifically made to fit your arms. You will probably be able to wear these only at night as they prevent you from cutting off circulation to your hands during sleep by bending your wrists or sleeping with your hands in funny positions.

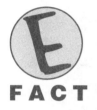

FACT

Your wrist splints should be long enough that you are supported for about three-fourths of the length of your forearm, and yet short enough that you can bend your elbow. Try the wrist splints on before buying them. If they are too short, they may only cause more problems with circulation.

Wrist and Hand Stretches

There are also several stretches that can be helpful in preventing hand and wrist problems. These stretches are designed to increase your circulation. You can do them several times a day, but it's very important that you do them prior to beginning your work and again as you take breaks. Also, remember that the longer you hold the stretches, the longer they will last. Try to figure that a ten-second stretch will last you about an hour whereas a thirty-second stretch will last you about three hours. These stretches need to be counted slowly, not as quickly as you can get to ten.

■ Finger Curl

Hold your left arm straight out in front of you, palm-side down. Place your right hand over the top of your left hand, again, palm-side down. Slowly curl the fingers of your right hand over those of your left hand. Encourage the left hand and fingers to curl as far under as possible.

You will feel that this stretches the muscles in the top of your forearm. Hold this stretch for ten to thirty seconds. Repeat this with your right hand.

■ Backward Finger Bend

Hold your left arm straight out in front of you, palm-side down. Place your right hand under the bottom of your left hand, palm-side up. Use the fingers of your right hand to press the fingers of your left hand upward, toward your body as far as you can comfortably go. Hold this stretch for ten to thirty seconds. Repeat this with your right hand.

■ Thumb Twists

Hold your left arm straight out in front of you, palm-side down. Use your right hand to grasp the thumb of your left hand. Rotate the left hand toward the floor as far as you can comfortably go. Hold this stretch for ten to thirty seconds. Repeat this with your right hand. In reverse thumb twists, hold your left arm straight out in front of you, palm-side down. Use your right hand to grasp the thumb of your left hand. Rotate the left hand toward the ceiling as far as you can comfortably go. Hold this stretch for ten to thirty seconds. Repeat this with your right hand.

Sample Arm-Specific Exercises

Exercises that work your arms, back, and shoulders can help you in your everyday life. Many are simple and require only a few repetitions to be effective.

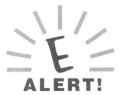
ALERT!

Doing arm exercises several times a week or having the movements incorporated into another form of exercise, such as aerobics, will enable you to receive the full benefits of the exercises you do.

Stretches

■ Arm Raise

While seated or standing, inhale and bring your arms over your head, keeping your elbows slightly bent. As you raise your arms, feel your spine loosen and lengthen. As you reach the peak, slowly straighten your elbows with your palms toward the ceiling (see **FIGURE 9-1**). Hold this pose for a few seconds and release slowly as you exhale. To steady yourself, try clasping your hands above your head. If your fingers or wrists feel stiff after doing this exercise, shake them very gently to release tension. Repeat this movement often to help release tension.

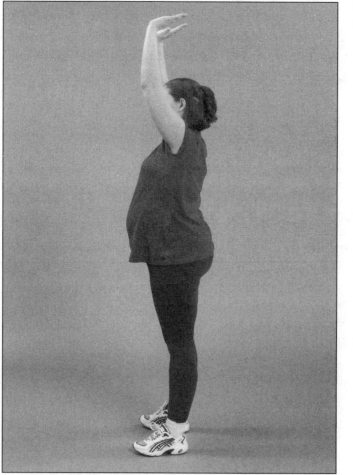

FIGURE 9-1
Arm Raise

■ Lat Stretch

Sit on the floor with a prop or blanket between your legs, supporting your weight. Rest backward toward your heels comfortably. Raise your right arm over your head, and bend it down toward your spine, behind your head. Stretch your fingers downward without straining. Allow the left arm to come up and hold your right elbow (see **FIGURE 9-2**). Without pulling, gently stretch the right arm toward the ceiling. Hold this pose for a count of five. This movement should not be bouncy or jerky, as this can hurt your arms. Repeat with your left arm. You may repeat this movement as often as you like.

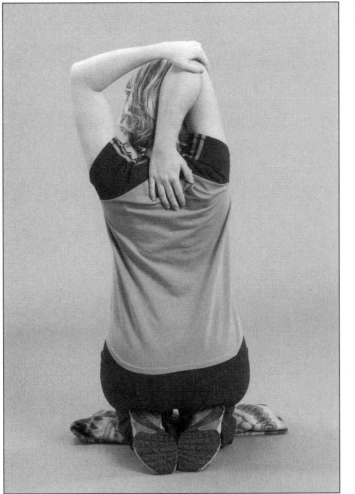

FIGURE 9-2
Lat Stretch

■ Kneeling Shoulder Stretch

Kneel on a soft surface on the floor facing a wall (use a towel if you need to), about a foot away from the wall. Spread your knees as far apart as you need to in order to allow your growing belly to rest comfortably on the floor. Turn your feet in toward the center, and drop the lower part of your pelvis, relaxing your pelvic floor as you do (see **FIGURE 9-3**). Raise your arms over your head with your palms facing the wall. Place your hands as high above your head on the wall as you can go without straining or causing yourself pain (see **FIGURE 9-4**). Consciously think of elongating your spine and relaxing backward onto your feet. Hold this stretch for ten seconds or more. Then release your arms slowly to your side and let your weight rest farther back on your feet.

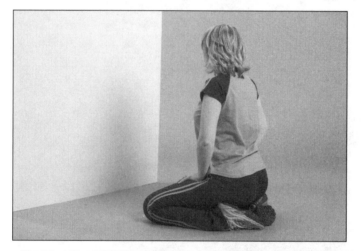

FIGURE 9-3
Kneeling Shoulder
Stretch

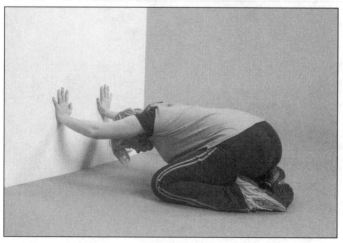

FIGURE 9-4
Let your head gently
lean forward and
feel the stretch
between your
shoulder blades and
in your upper arms.

■ Wall Pushups

Facing the wall, place your hands palm down on the wall, walk your feet backward, away from the wall (see **FIGURE 5-1**, p. 58). Slowly bend your elbows, bringing your upper body closer to the wall (see **FIGURE 5-2**, p. 58). Do about ten repetitions of the exercise. Remember to keep your spine in the proper alignment while doing this exercise.

■ Seated Pectoral Stretch

While tailor sitting on the floor or on a birth ball, place your hands on your lower back above your buttocks. Concentrate on pulling your shoulder blades together and continue breathing. Do this exercise ten times.

■ Posture Retraining

Place your back against the wall; slowly walk your feet forward until they are 6 to 8 inches in front of you. Press your glutes, shoulder blades, and the back of your head into the wall (see **FIGURE 5-3**, p. 59). Slowly raise your arms at a 90-degree angle, bent elbow to the wall, and press them to the wall as well. Slowly raise your arms, keeping them on the wall, above your head (see **FIGURE 5-4**, p. 59).

■ Chest Stretch

Stand with your feet hip-width apart. Take a step forward on either foot. As you inhale, extend your arms to your sides, the palms should be facing forward (see **FIGURE 6-3**, p. 79). Gently stretch back until you feel tension in your chest. If the intensity is too much or you are on bed rest, try doing this exercise in a chair or in your bed. Do several repetitions to help stretch the chest area.

Curls and Presses

■ Biceps Curl

Stand with soft knees shoulder-width apart. Pull in your abdominal muscles and lift your chest. Remember to keep your spine elongated. Tuck your elbows into your sides, forearms facing upward. Close your fists and slowly raise your fist to your chest. You can do this one arm at a time or two at a time. You should use your body as resistance at first.

Do this exercise ten times on each side to work your biceps. As you get stronger, you can add hand weights or dumbbells to increase resistance.

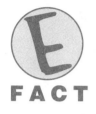

FACT

The average full-term baby will weigh about 7½ pounds at birth. While this sounds like a very little weight to have to carry around, the truth is that carrying around 7-plus pounds for more than about thirty minutes will cause your arms and back to ache and become very sore. Strong muscles will help alleviate this problem.

■ Bicep Curls

Stand with your feet shoulder-width apart and pointing forward so that you have a solid base. Take a weight and place it in your left hand (see **FIGURE 9-5**). Keep your left elbow close to your side, with your arm bent

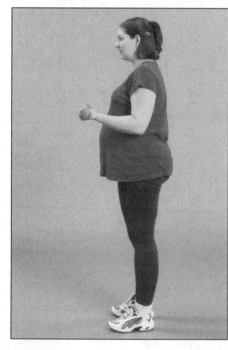

FIGURE 9-5
Bicep Curls

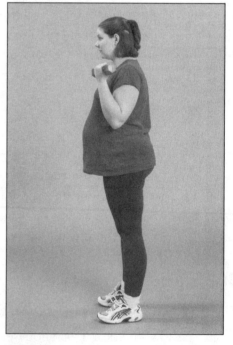

FIGURE 9-6
Avoid jerky movements as they can hurt you or cause you to let go of the weight.

parallel to the floor. Slowly raise the weight to about shoulder level (see **FIGURE 9-6**). Slowly lower the weight to the starting position. Do not go too quickly or use jerky movements. If you find yourself struggling or straining, use less weight. Repeat this exercise for eight to ten repetitions. Repeat on the opposite side. You can also do this in a seated position or without weights.

Exercise with Flex Bands

Flex bands are great for use with arm exercises. They allow you to exercise the arms without necessarily straining more. This is particularly true in the latter months of your pregnancy when some movements may be more difficult due to your increasing abdominal growth and the shift in your center of gravity.

■ Single Arm Lifts

Stand with one foot slightly forward, and your feet about shoulder-width apart. Stand on your flex band with your right foot, while grasping the other end of the band with your right hand (see **FIGURE 8-1**, p. 112). Palm down, slowly raise the right arm to shoulder level. Hold this pose for up to five seconds and slowly lower the right arm. Repeat this motion ten times. Then switch to your left arm for another ten repetitions.

■ Double Arm Lifts

Stand in the middle of your flex band. Hold one end of the band in each hand, while your arms hang by your sides. Relax and bend your knees slightly, while maintaining your spine in an upright position. Slowly, and together, raise both hands to your sides, palms upward, until you reach shoulder level. Be careful to use only your arms and not your shoulders in this exercise. The goal is to strengthen your arms to help you gain strength for tasks such as lifting your new baby. Do this exercise for ten repetitions.

■ Side Arm Stretches

Stand with your feet shoulder-width apart. Take the flex band in both hands, with your palms facing upward. Your arms and elbows should be tucked into your sides (see **FIGURE 9-7**). Hold the right hand steady as you move your left forearm and hand slowly away from your body (see **FIGURE 9-8**). When you reach your limit, slowly bring your left hand back to its starting position. Repeat this exercise ten times. Switch to exercising your right hand, while your left hand remains steady. Do another set of ten repetitions on that side.

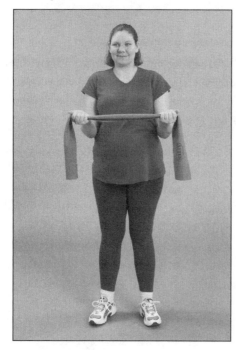

FIGURE 9-7
Side Arm Stretches

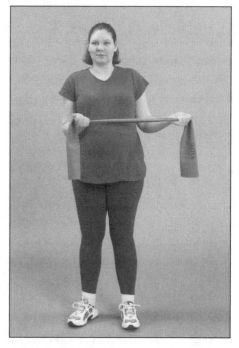

FIGURE 9-8
Remember to follow your natural range of motion to avoid hurting yourself.

Developing a Program of Exercises

What exercises you choose to do will help develop your muscles. Choosing them will depend on where you are starting at from a strength, flexibility, and tone standpoint. Do not be influenced by what others think you should be doing. Your arms will follow when you lead.

Look for areas that need your attention. Focus on where you have pain or tightness. Sometimes you go for the weak spots. The most important thing is a well-rounded workout for your arms. You don't want to overexercise certain parts while neglecting others. This can lead to more pain and trouble than you had to begin with! Always balance your arm work.

Using Weights for Arm Work

While weights are definitely not an absolute necessity, they can be very helpful in your arm fitness program. Simple resistance may not be enough for many women. This might be true for you if you have had a lot of exercise experience with your arms.

If you are more advanced in your arm work, bands might be only a temporary solution as you are getting back into your regular routine or if your pregnancy calls for cutting back on certain exercises.

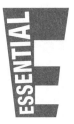

Avoid dropping your weights on the floor after use. You should set them down gently. This will not only avoid injuring yourself but will keep your equipment lasting longer

There is not one weight that is right or wrong for everyone. The best test of weight limit is your comfort level. Lifting weights should be a slight strain, but it should never feel overpowering. Lifting too much weight can damage your muscles so watching what you lift is important. Increase your weights gradually. Consider a personal training meeting if you have significant questions about weights. Remember, it is not a competition.

Chapter 10

Oh, Those Abdominals!

Pregnancy is obviously not the time to worry about a washboard stomach. Your six-pack abs will have to wait until after the birth of your baby. That said, there is still plenty that you can do to work your abdominal muscles during pregnancy without going overboard or injuring yourself.

Identifying Your Abdominal Muscles

Your abdominal muscles run from under your breastbone all the way to your pubic bone. This set of muscles is called the *rectus abdominis*. Underneath the rectus muscles are two sets of muscles that run at an angle toward the center of your abdomen, called your *obliques*. These muscles help you twist and turn and define your waist. The layer beneath the obliques is called the *transverses abdominis*. Running the entire length of your abdomen, this muscle supports your organs. It also covers a lot of area under your other muscles.

Abs Workout Positions

When exercising your abdominal muscles, it is important to note that the exercises are most effective on these muscles when you do them while lying on your back. During pregnancy lying flat on your back for vigorous exercise is not recommended after about sixteen weeks' gestation. Therefore, do your abdominal work in other positions, including all fours, standing, or sitting. You can also alternate a few back-lying (supine) exercises and a few non-supine.

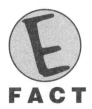

FACT

The size and shape of your belly will have no effect on your pregnancy or birth. There are plenty of people who try to predict the sex of your baby based on the shape of your belly or the size. These are all just myths. It is also not possible to determine how many babies are in your uterus simply by looking.

The Philosophy of Abs Work in Pregnancy

Popular literature used to say that you should never exercise your abdominal muscles during pregnancy because of a fear that it would harm your pregnancy or your baby. Today, we realize that these muscles are so important for pregnancy and beyond that we have had to rethink our teachings about abdominal exercise in pregnancy. The consensus is now that while it is safe to exercise your abdominal muscles during pregnancy, certain precautions must be taken.

Why the Abs Matter in Birth and Beyond

You might wonder why we bother talking about abdominal muscles during pregnancy if the benefits can't be seen or, supposedly, used during pregnancy. The point of exercising these muscles is that they will be used on a daily basis. Poor muscle tone in this area can lead to increased pregnancy complaints.

Back pain is one of the most common complaints of pregnancy. The surprising fact is that much of your back pain can have to do with your abdominal muscles. How strong and toned your abs are will dictate how well your back is supported. This is not to say that abs work is all you need to prevent back pain. Having an imbalance of either set of your muscles will cause you pain.

Labor

You know that your abdominal muscles support your internal organs, and this is true of the uterus as well. Your abdominal muscles will be busy at work during your labor, supporting your uterus as it contracts to open your cervix. By knowing these muscles well, you can help to keep them relaxed. This will help your baby enter your pelvis in a timely and efficient fashion, and therefore actually help speed labor along.

ESSENTIAL

If you are asked not to push for any reason during this second stage of labor, lift your chin from your chest and look upward. Begin to breathe lightly, as if imagining a feather is floating above your face. Breathe as if to keep that feather from falling to you. This will disengage your abdominal muscles and reduce the amount of pressure on the baby.

The position you choose in labor will help or hinder your process. By assuming upright positions you will help your baby enter the pelvis and apply more pressure on the cervix to help it dilate. Once you begin pushing, this upright position will allow you to use gravity to help you push your baby into the world as your body is aligned properly.

Once your cervix is fully dilated, you will begin to have the urge to push or bear down. It is during this portion of labor, known as the second stage of labor, that you will push your baby into the world. When you actively begin pushing, you will use your abdominals and your breathing, which is deeply related to your abdominal muscles, to help urge your baby into the world.

Assessing Your Abdominal Needs

Before any abdominal workout in pregnancy, it is important to know where you're starting from. If you had great abdominal muscles prior to pregnancy, you may worry about the loss of tone or definition. While it is true that your waist and abdomen do disappear during pregnancy, the muscles that you have attained are able to maintain tone and fitness, while providing you with a stable body.

If you've never really given your abdominal muscles much thought, now might be the time to start. An important first step is to recognize any problems you currently have with your abdominal muscles.

Diastasis Recti

It is highly recommended that you check your rectus muscles along the central seam, directly down the center of your abdominal muscle, for a separation, known as a diastasis recti. This condition can occur for many reasons, pregnancy being one of them. However, you can work on this diastasis recti during pregnancy to help lessen its effects and decrease the width.

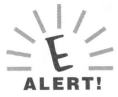

ALERT!

No matter what anyone tells you, the truth is that there is no cure or absolute prevention for stretch marks. A well-toned body, good nutritional status, and well-hydrated skin all help in the fight against stretch marks, although genetics will win every time. Avoid the magic cures that promise miracle cures or prevention treatment.

To check for the diastasis recti, begin by lying on your back with your knees bent. Slowly raise your head and shoulders, stretching your arms toward your knees. Place the fingers of one hand horizontally just above your belly button, in the center, near the seam of your muscles (see **FIGURE 10-1**). You will know you are in the right spot because you can feel the abdominal muscles tighten on each side. Make note of how many fingers fit in this area of separation.

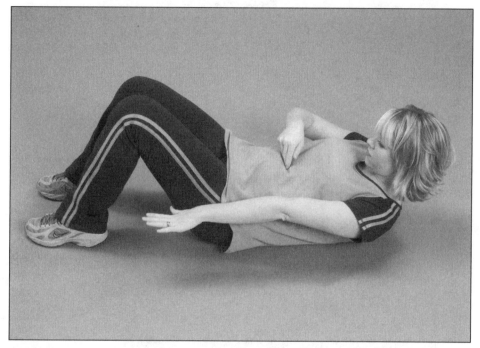

FIGURE 10-1
Checking for a separation of the diastasis recti.

It is perfectly normal to have a separation in these muscles during pregnancy. If you can fit three or more fingers in this pace, you need to do corrective exercises during pregnancy. These exercises are designed to help prevent this gap from growing.

The morning before you get out of bed and the evening before you go to sleep are the perfect times to do these brief exercises. Lie on your back with your knees drawn up. Cross your arms over your abdomen, grasping each side with the hand from the opposite side (see **FIGURE 10-2**). You will use your wrists or arms, depending on the size of your abdomen, to support your muscles as you slowly raise your head while you exhale. While you do this, gently pull your hands toward the center of your body (see **FIGURE 10-3**). This exercise should only be done a few times a day.

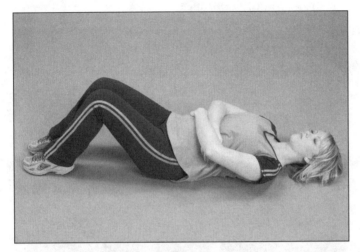

FIGURE 10-2
Resolving a separation of the diastasis recti.

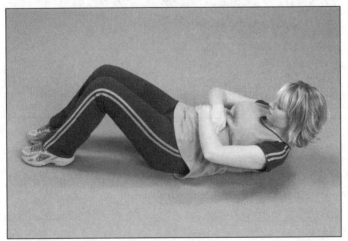

FIGURE 10-3
Remember, this is a gentle motion to help shorten the separation.

Know Your Absolute Limits

Your abdominal muscles are so important to your overall health and fitness level that it pays to really respect these muscles. Including some form of abs work in every workout can be very easy to do. However, remember to be wary of too much exercise or exercises that are too much for your stage of pregnancy.

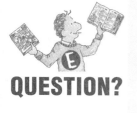

QUESTION?

Is it possible to have abdominal muscles that are too strong? If you have great abs prior to pregnancy, you may worry that your six-pack will prevent your body from growing and expanding as it should. It is important to note that this is not the case, and your baby will grow just fine. Be sure to check with your practitioner at every visit for an update of your uterine growth.

Abdominal Exercises for Everyone

Exercises for your abs may bring to mind hard workouts that leave you gasping for breath. The truth is that even the smallest exercise can have a lasting effect on your abdominal muscles. That said, exercising your abs should always be a part of your workout. There are abdominal exercises that can be done by everyone, including when you are very pregnant or newly postpartum.

Breathing

Your breath and breathing will be a very important key to many things in your pregnancy. Exercise and fitness are only the beginning of the need to be aware of your breath. Do not be tempted to ignore your breathing. It will be the key to relaxation in labor and will help you focus. It will help you to exercise and tone your muscles through appropriate concentration. It also tones your mind as well as your body.

Deep Breathing

Deep abdominal breathing sounds easy. The good news is that it is very easy. Learning to do true deep abdominal breathing while pregnant is simple, because you've got a great target—your baby. Sit in a tailor position and sit up with your spine as elongated as possible. Close your eyes and inhale very deeply. Imagine taking the air in and directing it toward your baby. If you have trouble breathing slowly, try counting your breaths. Slowly count to five as you inhale. Hold that breath for several seconds and then slowly release the breath for a count of five.

Stronger and Tighter Abs

Abdominal Strengthening

Sit on a birth ball with your feet about hip-distance apart. Sit up on the ball and elongate your spine (see **FIGURE 10-4**). You want to keep your

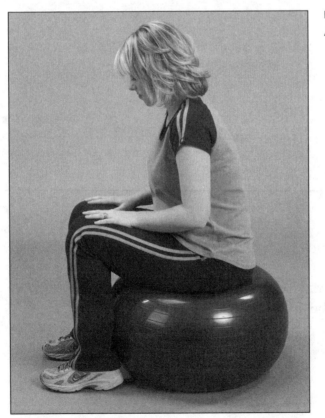

FIGURE 10-4
Abdominal Strengthening

spine elongated and pull your abdominal muscles in toward your belly button as you exhale. If it helps you, imagine coughing to find the abdominal muscles. Breathe normally as you do this exercise. Repeat the exercise ten times. This is an exercise that is appropriate for all phases of pregnancy and recovery. It is also great for beginning relaxation.

■ Abdominal Tightening

Seated on a birth ball, place your hands on your abdomen. Tilt your pelvis and as you inhale pull your abdominal muscles inward. Feel your abdomen move as your hands rest on them. Hold the pose for five seconds, while breathing. Repeat this exercise ten times.

Tilts, Curls, and More

■ Kneeling Abdominal Curl

Kneeling on the floor with your hands forward, palms down, tilt your pelvis in, pulling your baby toward the center of your body (see **FIGURE 7-10**, p. 104). Hold this pose for a count of ten. Repeat ten times. You can also do this by leaning across a chair to support your upper body.

■ Pelvic Rock/Pelvic Tilt

This is a hallmark pregnancy exercise. It provides so many benefits. You will see it mentioned in many categories because of its importance to your health and fitness status. The basic pelvic tilt is done on hands and knees, with your back straight, not sagging (see **FIGURE 5-7**, p. 61). Isolate your pelvis and tilt it toward your abdomen. As you do so, inhale and hold your breath to the count of five. Imagine pulling your abdominal muscles in at your belly button. Slowly release to a neutral position.

■ Side Bending (Tail Wagging)

This is a great exercise that can also provide you with a stretch. On hands and knees, with your back straight and not sagging, slowly pull your right hip toward your right shoulder (see **FIGURE 10-5**). The only part of your body that moves is your hips. Be sure to hold your shoulders and upper body still. Go as far as is comfortable for your body. Repeat this exercise ten times on each side. You can do these exercises one side at a time or alternate one side and then the next. To modify this exercise, try leaning over a chair or a birth ball to support your upper body. This is also a great exercise if you are having side pain.

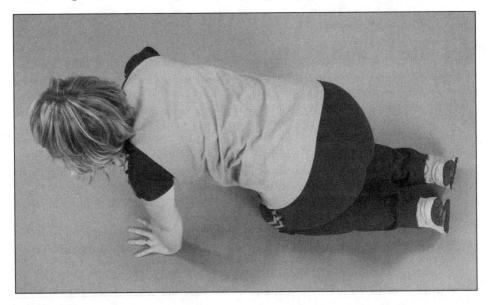

FIGURE 10-5
Side Bending (Tail Wagging)

First-Trimester Abdominal Exercises

Some exercises for your abdominal muscles are not appropriate for all phases of pregnancy. During the first trimester, little change has taken place to affect the abdominal muscles in your body. You are still able to lie freely on your back without compromising your body or baby, and without thinking about it.

Sample Abs Exercise Program

The following exercises can be done during the first trimester. Many can be adapted for your postpartum at a later date:

■ Heel Sliding

This exercise should only be done during the first trimester or during postpartum. You begin by lying on your back, knees up (see **FIGURE 10-6**). With your abdominal muscles pulled in toward your belly button, begin sliding your legs away from your body (see **FIGURE 10-7**). Stop before you need to move your spine. Slowly return your legs to the starting position. Repeat this exercise ten times.

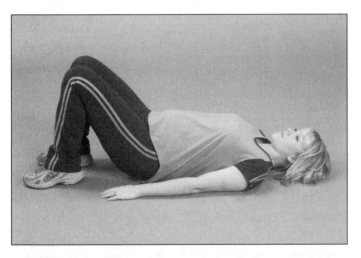

FIGURE 10-6
Heel Sliding

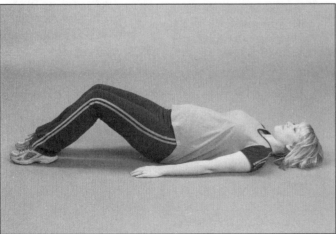

FIGURE 10-7
Remember, this is a gentle movement

■ Crunches

This exercise is best for the first trimester only. Lie down on your back with your knees bent. Your feet should be about hip-width apart and flat on the floor. Be sure your abdominal muscles are pulled in (see **FIGURE 10-8**). Doing a small pelvic tilt will help you achieve this effect. Place your hands on your upper legs. Slide your hands toward your knees as you slowly raise your head and shoulders off the floor (see **FIGURE 10-9**). This is not a huge movement and you should keep a space between your neck and chest. Breathing is essential; always remember to inhale as you release backward. The key to this abdominal exercise is a slow, steady pace. Jerky, bouncing movements will only cause you to injure yourself. You can do two or three sets of ten crunches.

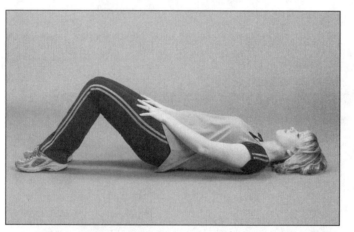

FIGURE 10-8
Crunches

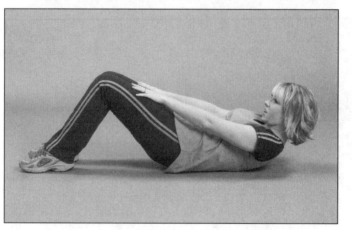

FIGURE 10-9
Remember to inhale as you release the hold.

Diagonal Curl-up

Lie down on your back with your spine elongated. Pull your knees up, feet hip-width apart and your feet flat on the floor. As you inhale, bring your left shoulder off the floor toward your right knee (see **FIGURE 10-10**). Be careful not to come farther than your shoulder blade. This does not provide you with any more exercise, as at this point you cease using your abdominal muscles. Exhale and slowly lie back. Switch sides, bringing your right shoulder toward your left knee. Repeat ten times for each side.

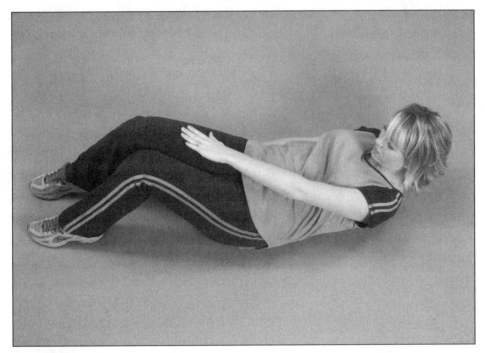

FIGURE 10-10
Diagonal Curl-up

■ Abdominal Stabilization

You will need your birth ball to aid you in this exercise. Lie down on your back, while placing your calves and feet on the birth ball. For support, place your hands at your sides. As you contract your abdominal muscles and your buttocks, lift your lower body from the floor (see **FIGURE 10-11**). Press your feet and calves into the ball to prevent it from rolling around. Hold this pose for a few seconds and then slowly lower your body back to the floor. Breathe normally and repeat ten times.

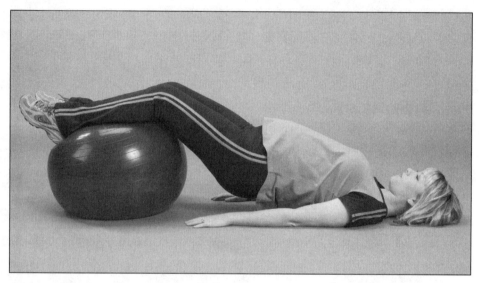

FIGURE 10-11
Abdominal Stabilization on the Ball

The Benefits

So when exercising your abdominal muscles, remember that the benefits will affect everything from your posture and how you move each day to the birth of your baby. It will even affect how quickly you recover after the birth of your baby. Remember to check for separation of the rectus muscles and alternate your supine positions with other positions to avoid maternal supine hypotension syndrome. With hard work and dedication, it will pay off. The results will be an amazing middle section! Ⓔ

Chapter 11

Y **Lean Legs and Strong Glutes**

Your legs and glutes are very important parts of your body. You use them on a daily basis to stand, walk, lift, and bend. Strong legs and glutes also give you an advantage when it is time to give birth. You will use them to position yourself comfortably for labor and then for birth. By increasing the strength and tone during pregnancy, you help make this part of labor much easier.

Identifying Leg and Glute Muscles

Your legs and glutes are the largest muscle groups in your body. They help you walk, bend, lift your legs, stabilize your body, and promote your back health. It is important to know something about these muscles as you exercise them. Being able to visualize where they are and how they work will make your workouts more effective.

Hip Flexors and Quadriceps

The hip flexors assist you in lifting your legs to the front. You use these muscles while walking up stairs or standing up on a step. They are located opposite of your glutes. If you sit a lot during the day, they may be shorter than normal. Exercise and stretching can help strengthen them so that they are more useful.

Your quadriceps are located in the front of your thighs. As you can see by the prefix *quad*, there are four main muscles in this group:

- Rectus femoris (the largest)
- Vastus medialis
- Vastus lateralis
- Vastus intermedius

The main function of this muscle group is to allow you to extend your leg from the knee, as in walking or bending.

Glutes (Buttocks)

Your buttocks are often referred to as your "glutes." This is actually a group of three muscles: gluteus maximus (the largest), gluteus medius, and gluteus minimus (smallest).

The gluteus maximus helps you walk and jump. The gluteus medius helps with more lateral movement. The gluteus minimus is used to help rotate the leg outward. It is also located underneath the area where, one might say, you have saddlebags.

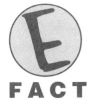

The more strengthened a muscle is, the more calories it burns at rest. So even if you are sleeping, muscle mass will be burning calories. Fatty tissue does not do this even while you exercise. So the more muscles you have, the more calories you burn at rest.

Thighs and Hamstrings

A special word needs to be said about your thighs, particularly your inner thighs. This area is one of the least worked areas of the body. And yet, it is also the one that will be called upon repeatedly in labor.

The inner thigh is called your hip adductor. It helps move your legs across the body, for example, in crossing your feet over each other, or doing dance steps. It also helps stabilize your knees. The outer thigh is called your hip abductor. This muscle helps move your foot away from your body and helps in stabilizing your hips and knees.

The easiest way to remember the difference in their functions is to look at the prefix. To add to the body is to be a hip adductor—you are moving that leg inward, toward your body. The abductor moves away from the body.

The hamstrings are located in the back of your thighs. They function to bring your heel toward your glutes and to help you bend your knees. They do work with the other muscles in this area to produce a movement, such as bringing your leg up behind you. Many women find this area to be a tight area, which can cause pain. Stretching and warming up before a workout can help alleviate this problem.

Lower Leg

The calf muscles are located in the back of your leg, below the knee. The soleus and gastrocnemius muscles make up this muscle group. The soleus muscle lies underneath the gastrocnemius muscle, which is what you see when you look at your calf. These muscles help you stabilize the ankle joint and move when you lift your heel.

Your anterior tibialis, or shin muscle, is on the front part of your lower leg, under your knee. Unless you are suffering from shin splints, you probably don't pay much attention to this muscle, which is contracted as you lift the ball of your foot.

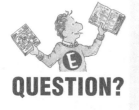

QUESTION?

How can I prevent leg cramps at night?
Many pregnant women suffer from leg cramps, particularly at night. Well-toned and strengthened muscles will be less susceptible to this problem, which can be very painful. Stretching the lower leg just before bed and ensuring that you have plenty of calcium and potassium in your diet are ways to help alleviate this problem.

Leg Muscles Are Key in Labor

When you think of labor, you probably have a television version in your mind. You might envision contractions and bed rest, coupled with funny breathing and screaming nasty things at those around you. Labor is much more than what you're shown on television. It's a combination of physical, mental, and emotional work.

During labor, it's clear that your uterus and abdominal muscles are working. What most pregnant women do not realize, however, is that their legs do a lot of work as well. We have learned about different positions that can be used to help facilitate an easier labor. Many of these positions require strong leg muscles to help support your body.

The Role They Play

During labor, your legs will carry you as you walk around to facilitate labor's progress. Your legs will help you assume positions to encourage your baby's descent into the birth canal. They will rock you in a chair and carry you to the shower or bathtub.

You will actually use your legs to assist you in pushing. While you won't actively push with your legs, you will have to hold them in different positions and use their force to assist you. Having strong muscles that are stretched and ready to go will be most beneficial. Using the muscles during pregnancy and actively preparing them for birth will give you the added benefit of stamina during labor.

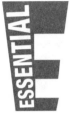

Squatting, which really requires practice and leg strength, opens your pelvic outlet by an additional 10 percent. This position facilitates the birth of your baby and is often jokingly called the midwives' forceps. Practicing this position during pregnancy will help you to use it more effectively during birth. It also helps prevent the need for episiotomy and/or tearing of the perineum.

While you are in labor and you come to the second stage, or pushing phase of labor, you can also enlist the help of others around you in holding your legs in certain positions. While you can't get a lot of leg support while squatting, your partner, doula, or nurses can help hold up your body. They can also help hold your legs, particularly if you are very tired or have had epidural anesthesia.

Basically, any fitness program you do should include leg work. Both your legs and glutes will play an important part in your labor and recovery. They will also help you recover more quickly once your baby is born.

Leg Exercises for Strength and Tone

The good news about working out your lower extremities during pregnancy is that there are very few contraindications to these exercises. The majority are simple to do and can be done nearly anywhere, at any time. There are very few modifications needed because of your pregnancy.

Since these areas make up a large portion of your muscle mass, remember that they need attention, too. Everyday exercises (for example, walking) do help this area, but you need to make a concerted effort to strengthen the legs and glutes.

Exercises for Hips, Buttocks, and Thighs

■ Lunge

Stand up without the support of the wall. Maintain the proper posture, while stepping back with your left leg. Your upper body should remain facing forward and not moving. Be sure to keep your right knee above your right ankle, as leaning or twisting could cause injury (see **FIGURE 5-5**, p. 60). Lower your body until your right thigh is nearly parallel to the floor. Raise your body by pressing into your right foot (see **FIGURE 5-6**, p. 60). Do about ten repetitions of this exercise and then repeat on the opposite side.

■ Squat

This can help strengthen the muscles of your thighs to allow for an easier time at birth if you choose to give birth in this position. Start by using a chair, or a partner, and stand facing him with your feet shoulder-width apart. Slowly lower your body, as he lowers his. Go down as far as you can, while keeping your heels on the floor (see **FIGURE 5-9**, p. 62). You will probably require some practice doing this exercise until you can do it alone and go down into a near-sitting position. Do ten squats, holding each one five to ten seconds. Avoid bouncing in between squats.

■ Supported Squat (Wall Squat) with the Ball

Standing up straight with your back facing a wall, place the birth ball between you and the wall around the center of your back and press it into the wall using your back. Slowly walk your feet forward, leaning back into the ball for support (see **FIGURE 7-6**, p. 102). As you walk forward, the ball will roll up to the center of your back, between your shoulder blades. This allows you to do a squat without having to worry about being steady or having a partner (see **FIGURE 7-7**, p. 102). When you are down as far as you can go, hold the pose for up to ten seconds, then slowly walk your feet back to their starting position allowing the ball to roll back to the center of your lower back.

■ Side Lying Stretches

Lying on your right side, stretch your right arm over your body as if reaching for something above your head. Focus on extending the arm as well at the leg and body (see **FIGURE 5-14**, p. 65). This should feel like a good tension release. Hold this pose for about ten seconds. Repeat on the left side.

■ Seated Leg Lifts

Sit on the edge of your bed or chair. Allow both of your feet to hang over the side. It is not necessary that your legs touch the ground. Drape the sock weight over your right ankle. Slowly raise the left leg as you exhale (see **FIGURE 11-1**). Do not bring your leg up to the point of pain, and it should not be raised higher than knee level. Slowly lower your leg. Repeat this for a count of ten repetitions on each leg.

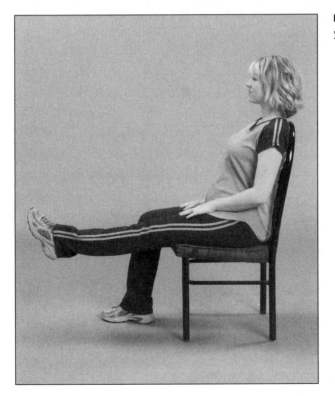

FIGURE 11-1
Seated Leg Lifts

■ Standing Leg Lifts

Stand with your hand on the wall or a chair for support. With your toes facing forward, lift the leg that is opposite the chair or the wall (see **FIGURE 11-2**). Lift it as high as you can without causing pain or losing your balance. Repeat this eight to ten times and then repeat on the opposite side.

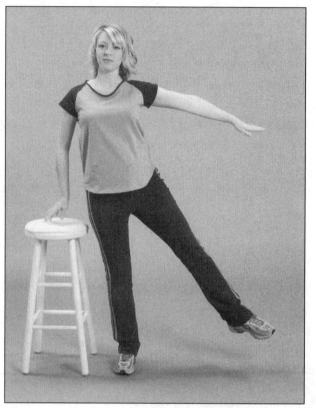

FIGURE 11-2
Standing Leg Lifts

Exercises for Your Lower Legs

There are not many exercises that fall into this category. But they are very effective at what they do. To increase the difficulty of these exercises, try adding a platform, like a book or even an aerobics step.

■ Heel Raises

Lean on a wall, facing the wall. Hold the wall with the palms of your hands. Extend your feet, raising your heels, like standing on the tip of your toes. Do this eight to ten times and repeat with the other foot.

■ Toe Raises

Stand facing a wall or a chair, using your hands for support. Take a slight step forward with your right foot. Place the weight of your body on the heel. Slowly raise your toes, like you are tapping them (see **FIGURE 11-3**). This should be a slow, controlled movement so you don't injure the muscles involved. Tap your toes slowly, eight to ten times, pausing at the peak to hold your foot up. Be sure to repeat this on the opposite foot.

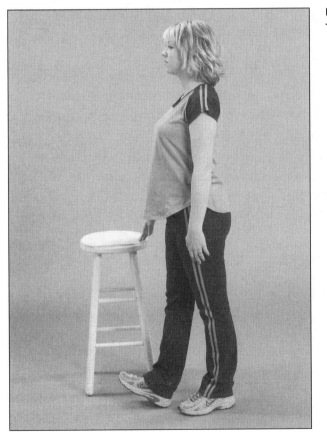

FIGURE 11-3
Toe Raises

■ Heel Extensions

Standing with your feet shoulder-width apart and your hands on your hips, bend your right knee and straighten that leg out to the front, with your left knee soft. Touch your right heel to the floor and return to standing. As you move your feet, raise your arms over your head, returning them to your hips as you bring your feet back to the beginning pose. Repeat this exercise ten times on each side. If you need a lower intensity, keep your hands on your hips rather than raise them over your head.

The Role of Glutes in Pregnancy

Pregnancy is the perfect time to tone your legs and bottom. It can help you identify different muscle groups and identify potential problem areas. It also gives you an advantage in labor as you prepare your body for the hard work of giving birth.

You do need to realize that your gluteal area is an area that is designed to accumulate fat deposits during pregnancy. This is your body's way of protecting you and your baby after birth should you need the extra fuel for feeding your baby. Breastfeeding and exercise are the best ways to remove this added fat on your body. So don't be concerned as your pregnancy progresses if you notice fat deposits being laid down in this area. It is not a sign that your workout efforts are failing. It is a sign that your body is doing an excellent job of preparing for your new baby.

Exercises to Strengthen Your Glutes

■ Pelvic Rock/ Pelvic Tilt

This is the perfect exercise for backache in pregnancy. It will not only help prevent them, but cure them as well. Assume an all-fours position, on your hands and knees. Think of holding your back in its natural alignment (see **FIGURE 5-7**, p. 61). Then tuck only your pelvis in, bringing your pubic bone toward your neck. Be sure to move only your pelvis (see **FIGURE 5-8**, p. 61). If it helps, have someone hold your pelvis so that you can learn to isolate this area. Later, this exercise can be done in different positions. You need to do two sets of twenty repetitions of the pelvic tilts. For an added bonus, do another set of twenty repetitions just before bed to help you sleep.

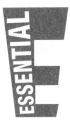

The pelvic rock or tilt can become your best friend. You can learn to do it standing up, while leaning against a wall for added comfort. In fact, if you take a canister of unopened tennis balls and place it behind the small of your back prior to doing the pelvic rocks, you can manage to give yourself a quick massage.

■ Lunge

Stand up without the support of the wall. Maintain the proper posture, while stepping back with your left leg. Your upper body should remain facing forward and not moving. Be sure to keep your right knee above your right ankle, as leaning or twisting could cause injury (see **FIGURE 5-5**, p. 60). Lower your body until your right thigh is nearly parallel to the floor. Raise your body by pressing into your right foot (see **FIGURE 5-6**, p. 60). Do about ten repetitions of this exercise and then repeat on the opposite side.

■ Squat

This can help strengthen the muscles of your thighs to allow for an easier time at birth if you choose to give birth in this position. Start by using a chair or a partner and stand facing him with your feet shoulder-width apart. Slowly lower your body, as he lowers his. Go down as far as you can, while keeping your heels on the floor (see **FIGURE 5-9**, p. 62). You will probably require some practice doing this exercise until you can do it alone and go down into a near-sitting position. Do ten squats, holding each for five to ten seconds. Avoid bouncing in between squats.

■ Supported Squat (Wall Squat)

Standing up straight with your back facing a wall, place the birth ball between you and the wall around the center of your back and press it into the wall using your back. Slowly walk your feet forward, leaning back into the ball for support (see **FIGURE 7-6**, p. 102). As you walk forward, the ball will roll up to the center of your back, between your shoulder blades. This allows you to do a squat without having to worry about being steady or having a partner (see **FIGURE 7-7**, p. 102). When you are down as far as you can go, hold the pose for up to ten seconds, then slowly walk your feet back to their starting position allowing the ball to roll back to the center of your lower back.

■ Leg Extensions

Sit on the edge of a chair. Use a dumbbell as a weight. Place it between your feet. Hold on to the edges of the chair and begin to raise your legs slowly, bringing the dumbbell with you. This will strengthen and flex your quads and glutes. Slowly return to your starting position. Repeat this exercise ten times. Be careful not to use too great a weight or to go too quickly.

Exercises for Those Who Sit

If you find yourself sitting at a desk all day, you may not feel like you're getting your legs stretched and exercised. You might even suffer from pain or swelling in the legs. To minimize the pain and swelling associated with pregnancy, be sure to drink plenty of water, stretch your legs often, and do focus at least some of your fitness time on your legs.

During the workday you may want to walk around a bit more to ensure good circulation. Rather than letting work pile up before you distribute it, consider making several trips as the work comes across your desk. Sure, you might walk to the copier two or three times more than you might before, but it will help your legs and body feel better during the day. Take the stairs when appropriate and walk around your neighborhood. Do whatever it takes to keep your legs moving!

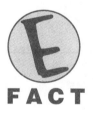

FACT

Varicose veins in the leg are not uncommon in pregnancy. If you find yourself with distended veins, be sure to show them to your doctor or midwife. You may need to wear support hose to help alleviate the problem. Elevating your feet above your heart also helps improve circulation. Watch for hot or painful spots, as it may indicate a blood clot. Let your practitioner know about this symptom right away.

Exercising your legs and bottom is very important. It can be so easy to focus on other areas during pregnancy. The benefits you will get from the exercise you do now will follow you to birth. This will also help make weight loss easier once your baby has been born. Ⓔ

Chapter 12

Weight Training
in Pregnancy

Weight training in pregnancy is an effective way to exercise. It will help you increase your strength and flexibility. It should be done two to three times per week in addition to other types of exercise. The purpose is to gain strength, using weights to help you achieve this goal. With a few small modifications, it is not only safe but also enjoyable for pregnancy.

Weightlifting Benefits

Weightlifting isn't about bulking up, nor is it about seeing who can lift how much. During pregnancy, the goal of weight training will be to work every major muscle group during your routine. Here are some benefits to lifting weights during pregnancy:

- Muscle burns more calories at rest than fat.
- Effective exercises of weightlifting require less time than other types of exercise.
- Weight training helps prevent osteoporosis by building bone.
- It reduces stress levels.
- Weight training increases energy levels and strength.
- It aids in rest and sleep.
- Strength training improves posture, balance, and joint stability.

Many people don't even realize that weightlifting is appropriate in pregnancy. In an ideal world, weight or strength training would be done two to three times per week. During pregnancy, weightlifting is perfectly acceptable with a few small limitations.

Safety Precautions

Weight training done in pregnancy is a perfectly acceptable form of exercise. Using the weight training to counterbalance the changes in your pregnant body can be very beneficial. There are just a few small tips to keep your workout safe and healthy for you and your baby.

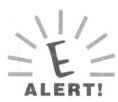

ALERT!

While you may be worried about weight training in your pregnancy, most women are able to maintain near the same weight-bearing intensity as they had achieved prior to pregnancy, though there can be a higher risk of injury if you're not careful.

Watch Your Posture

The first key to a safe pregnancy weight-training session is to be very aware of your posture. You want to be sure always to be cognizant of how you are holding your body. Your spine should be neutral; you should look forward. Hold your shoulders up and slightly back. This posture awareness will not only help you do the exercises more efficiently, but it will help protect you from injury.

Keep Your Knees Soft

Your knees should be kept soft. This means that you should not stand with your knees locked in one position. If you were to keep your knees locked, you would run the risk of injuring your knees or even passing out! So, watch those knees and remember to check for a bit of give.

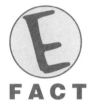

FACT

Your range of motion, how far you can safely move a joint, will also be affected by pregnancy and its associated hormones. Be sure to watch this as you exercise. This is true even of the simplest movements. If you experience pain or tenderness, do not repeat a certain exercise, or look at your overall positioning.

Contract Abdominal Muscles

Your abdominal muscles should be contracted while you are doing your workout. This is to help protect these muscles while you bear the weight of the exercises you are doing. It's also good practice for the rest of your life!

On exertion, you should also remember to pull in your Kegel muscles. This helps protect the pelvic floor. It's also a great way to remind you to fit your Kegel exercises in. After a while, this Kegel exercise becomes automatic any time you lift anything, whether that is your baby, your laundry, or anything else.

Rest and Stretch

Because of the added strain on your pregnant body from hormones, postural changes, and just general fatigue, you will definitely want to utilize a rest period of twenty-four hours between each workout session. Allowing your muscles to rest in between will give you a better workout with less risk of injury during your next session. You should also stretch between each group of exercises.

Watching Your Breathing While Lifting

As with every aspect of pregnancy, breathing is very important to your weightlifting routine. You must always keep in mind that as you breathe, you are taking in clean air for your baby. This oxygen nourishes your little one. It also helps make for a better workout for you. As you exhale, you actually detoxify your body. This is done by exhaling carbon dioxide from your body. You also take in air for your body to use to feel good.

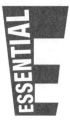

Remember that breathing during exercise is very important. If you find yourself having trouble remembering to breathe, always think of breathing specifically for your baby. This often helps moms remember to breathe.

Breath Holding

When exercising and lifting weights, you might have a picture in your mind of a typical weight lifter. This weight lifter might be holding her breath and turning red as she strains. This is absolutely not appropriate during pregnancy. This breath holding can be problematic in that it can cause problems with blood flow and oxygenation of your body and, therefore, your baby's body as well. It can also cause increased abdominal pressure. This is particularly true of prolonged breath holding.

Valsalva Maneuver

Another breathing technique you should not use when pregnant is called the Valsalva maneuver. This involves forcefully exhaling air while not releasing air from your lungs. This is much like breathing during a bowel movement. It can change your intra-abdominal pressure and cause problems for your pregnancy. So while lifting, remember to inhale and exhale on a regular basis.

Breathing Consciously

The key to breathing during weight or strength training is to breathe consciously. Eventually, you will not have to focus on your breathing as much as you will in the beginning. Always exhale on exertion. That's easy to remember because you will E (exhale) on E (exertion). Inhale as you lower the weights or return to a neutral pose.

Your breathing for relaxation may work really well. In addition, it teaches your body and reinforces that physical exertion can be accompanied by slow-paced breathing. It also helps oxygenate your body appropriately for the workout.

Safe Workout Tips

While there is not one safe workout that is appropriate for strength/weight training during pregnancy, there are basic guidelines to help you keep your workouts safe. When planning your workouts, keep the few simple rules in mind. That is always your best bet. Remember, you'll have days when you go full force and others when you need to take it easy. Always follow your body's lead.

Take Your Time

Time constraints make us hurry. This is true in everyday life as well as exercise. However, rushing your exercise routine, particularly weight training, can be very dangerous. Remember that a rushed workout is not the best workout. Take your time. Do your repetitions of exercises correctly and slowly. Really work the muscles. Doing a fast workout only increases your risk of injury.

Make Sure Technique Is Correct

Part of taking your time will be to watch your form. Watching your form and your technique will also alleviate many of the injuries associated with weight training. If you are not sure of the proper technique for a certain exercise, avoid it until you can receive some instruction. This also applies to finding a new way to modify an exercise because of pregnancy.

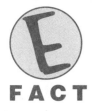

FACT

Lifting too much weight at once, or using improper form, is the fastest way to injure yourself during pregnancy or at any time. When you do get injured during your workout, it takes your body longer to heal because your body would rather devote its time and attention to growing a strong, healthy baby. This leaves you hurting and unable to exercise.

When using weights, remember always to use them the way they are supposed to be used. Again, if you don't know how to use the weights, wait for someone to help you. Try lighter weights the further you get into your pregnancy. You can always add more repetitions or sets to your workout. This also helps prevent injury to your muscles.

Use Good Judgment

During the third trimester, it may be better to switch to machines rather than free weights. The risk of injuring yourself is greater with free weights, particularly the further along you are in your pregnancy. Some trainers fear that using free weights will enable you to injure yourself by actually hitting your abdomen. If this concerns you at any point, move to the machines.

If you feel off balance or like you are having trouble with weightlifting, particularly with the upper body, try modifying these exercises. The easiest way to modify the upper body exercises is to use a sitting or other upright position rather than standing. You can do nearly all of your chest, arm, back, or shoulder lifts while seated. This is also true of many leg exercises.

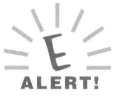

ALERT!

Seeing spots should never happen when you exercise. This is a sign that something is wrong. This can happen if your blood pressure is rising to dangerously high levels or falling to dangerously low levels. It also happens when you lift too much weight at once. If you ever find yourself seeing spots—stop immediately and ask for help. Call your midwife or doctor if the spots continue and definitely mention them at your next appointment.

Weight-Training Exercises

Weight training is not something to take lightly, no pun intended. You should seriously consider getting some professional, or at least experienced, help while exercising with weights. This is to help you prevent injury to you or your pregnancy, and to give you a good idea of what your body can handle.

Sample Exercise Program

There are some specific exercises that are routinely used by pregnant women of varying fitness levels that you might find helpful. You can do the majority of the following exercises using your body as a weight. If you need more resistance, use free weights or other equipment to help increase the difficulty level of the exercise.

■ Posture Retraining

Place your back against the wall; slowly walk your feet forward until they are 6 to 8 inches in front of you. Press your glutes, shoulder blades, and the back of your head into the wall (see **FIGURE 5-3**, p. 59). Slowly raise your arms at a 90-degree angle, bent elbows to the wall, and press them to the wall as well. Slowly raise your arms, keeping them on the wall, above your head (see **FIGURE 5-4**, p. 59).

■ Wall Pushups

Facing the wall, place your hands palm down on the wall, walk your feet backward, away from the wall (see **FIGURE 5-1**, p. 58). Slowly bend your elbows bringing your upper body closer to the wall (see **FIGURE 5-2**, p. 58). Do about ten repetitions of the exercise. Remember to keep your spine in the proper alignment while doing this exercise.

■ Biceps Curl

Stand with soft knees, shoulder-width apart. Pull in your abdominal muscles and lift your chest. Remember to keep your spine elongated. Tuck your elbows into your sides, forearms facing upward. Close your fists and slowly raise your fist to your chest. You can do this one arm at a time or two at a time. You should use your body as resistance at first. Do this exercise ten times on each side to work your biceps. As you get stronger, you can add hand weights or dumbbells to increase resistance.

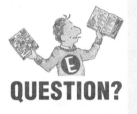

QUESTION?

What benefits do I get from weight or strength training postpartum?
Actually, you will get all of the same benefits of weight training that you get during pregnancy. The biggest advantage to doing postpartum weight training is that you will help reduce the amount of post-baby flab you find on your body. This is a source of stress for many women.

■ Wall Butterfly

Lie down on the floor with your bottom and feet against the wall, keep your soles together, and let your knees drop open. Use your hands to press your knees downward toward the wall (see **FIGURE 15-3**, p. 200). This will open up your pelvic area and strengthens your legs, inner thighs, and lower spine.

■ Hip Abduction Lying

Lie down on your back with your knees bent, feet flat on the floor, and your shoulders and hips firmly on the floor. Place your right ankle on your left knee. Bring your left knee toward your chest by grabbing your left thigh with your left hand (see **FIGURE 5-11**, p. 63). Hold this for about five seconds. Repeat on the opposite side.

■ Lunge

Stand up without the support of the wall. Maintain the proper posture, while stepping back with your left leg. Your upper body should remain facing forward and not moving. Be sure to keep your right knee above your right ankle, as leaning or twisting could cause injury (see **FIGURE 5-5**, p. 60). Lower your body until your right thigh is nearly parallel to the floor. Raise your body by pressing into your right foot (see **FIGURE 5-6**, p. 60). Do about ten repetitions of this exercise and then repeat on the opposite side.

■ Military Press

Sit on the edge of a chair or bench with your feet about hip-width apart. Your knees should be bent with your feet flat on the floor. Using a dumbbell in each hand, face your palms inward. Lift your arms above shoulder level, slowly and steadily. Then bring them back to their starting position at your sides. Repeat this exercise for ten repetitions.

Flex Band Use

Flex bands are great for weight training in pregnancy. They are portable and cost effective. They also allow you to choose the amount of resistance you require for any given exercise. Flex bands also carry little potential for injury to your or your baby during pregnancy.

Sample Flex Band Exercises

■ Single Arm Lifts

Stand with one foot slightly forward, and your feet about shoulder-width apart. Stand on your flex band with your right foot, while grasping the other end of the band with your right hand (see **FIGURE 8-1**, p. 112). Palm down, slowly raise the right arm to shoulder level (see **FIGURE 8-2**, p. 112).

Hold this pose for up to five seconds and slowly lower the right arm. Repeat this motion ten times. Then switch to the left arm.

Side Arm Stretches

Stand with your feet shoulder-width apart. Take the flex band in both hands, with your palms facing upward. Your arms and elbows should be tucked into your sides (see **FIGURE 9-7**, p. 136). Hold the left hand steady as you move the right forearm and hand slowly away from your body (see **FIGURE 9-8**, p. 136). Follow your natural range of motion here, and don't overdo it. When you reach your limit, slowly bring your right hand back to its starting position. Repeat this exercise ten times. Switch to your left hand moving while your right hand remains steady.

Seated Row

Sitting on the floor with a flex band wrapped around your feet at the middle of the band, hold one end of the band in each hand (see **FIGURE 6-9**, p. 84). Your palms should be facing the floor. Pull the bands to your chest. Hold this for one count. Slowly release the tension in the band, returning to the original pose. Repeat this rowing motion ten times.

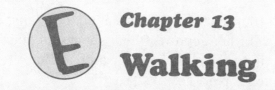

Chapter 13

Walking

Walking is something you do every day without giving it much thought. Walking is a great aerobic exercise that can be adapted to pregnancy. This form of exercise can provide you with a great cardiovascular workout. Walking is also one of the best exercises to do for beginning exercisers; nearly everyone can walk, no matter what their pregnancy or fitness status. It is also easily adaptable to any lifestyle including that of life with your new baby.

Getting Started

Walking is great, even if you have not exercised before. This, however, does not mean that you should run right out and walk around your neighborhood three times today. Any form of exercise in pregnancy requires more thought than that. This is particularly true if you have not been exercising before.

Once you have talked to your doctor or midwife about beginning a walking program and have his or her approval, think about your fitness levels. If you are moderately fit, you can probably begin by doing a ten-minute walk, three or more times per week.

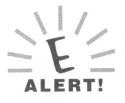

ALERT!

When considering walking in pregnancy, the key is to listen to your body. While it is a great exercise, you do need to talk to your doctor or midwife about the benefits and risks to your health, your baby's, and your pregnancy. Be sure to be prepared for all of the changes in your body.

From the ten-minute walk, you would move to adding a minute or two, once a week, until you had reached about a thirty-minute walk. If the thirty-minute walk is not strenuous enough for you, try adding your arms to the mix. By pumping your arms up and down while you walk, you are adding more aerobic energy to the mix.

Fitness Walking Precautions

While walking may be something you do every day, walking for fitness does have some things to watch for. Common mistakes are made that can harm you or cause you to lose your balance more easily. Be sure to keep these things in mind.

Proper Posture

Watching your posture is key, as with any exercise. Be sure to tuck your pelvis inward, rather than allow your back to hollow out. This poor posture can intensify back strain and cause fatigue and soreness. Try to imagine a string pulling your head up from the neck. Allow your spine to follow as you walk. Much like keeping the proverbial book balanced on your head, your walking posture needs to be prim and proper to avoid difficulties.

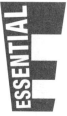

You should not watch your feet while walking. When you do this, you tend to lean forward. This posture can cause you to round your shoulders, leading with your head and neck. It can also exaggerate your waddle. Your feet should come out in front, from the hip. When you watch your feet, you tend to rotate them slightly differently.

Invest in Comfortable Walking Shoes

The proper shoes are also very important when walking. You may choose to just use your athletic shoes, but if you start to put any mileage on your feet with walking, you will notice that your feet are not very forgiving. For this reason, it is recommended that you invest in a pair of shoes that you use simply for walking and other forms of exercise. Go to a sporting goods store and allow the salespeople to help you find the shoe that is right for you. Use these shoes only when you exercise, as it will prolong their life and your budget.

Exhaustion and Overheating

Your exertion needs to be monitored, as with any form of exercise. You will want to avoid becoming too exhausted. If you begin to feel winded, remember the talk test: Could you still carry on a conversation without gasping for breath? If the answer is no, stop what you are doing and rest before heading back home.

Overheating can also be a problem. This is true, even in cold weather. Be sure to dress in layers. This allows you to remove a layer of clothing if you need to do so. If it is cold outside, dress one layer warmer than you think you might need. This will allow you to remove a layer as you begin to warm up from walking.

You will also want to be sure that your clothing is loose. As your belly expands, wearing your partner's sweats, or specific maternity jogging pants or exercise pants may be a must. This will also help prevent overheating. Check the fabric—some might even provide wicking, pulling water away from your skin as you sweat.

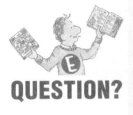

QUESTION?

What should my heart rate be?
Your target heart rate is calculated by subtracting your age from 220. You want to be between 65 and 85 percent of that number. For example, if you are 30, your maximum heart rate is 190. Multiply that by .65, and then .85, and your target range would be 123 to 161.

Walking Stretches

Stretching is important both before and after your walk, so always make time to stretch. Remember also that the warmup and cool-down periods are the keys to a healthy workout. Here are some sample walking stretches you can do before and after your walking workout.

■ Neck Stretch

Stand with your feet shoulder-width apart. Let your shoulders be held up and back. The crown of your head should be pulling upward. Slowly let your chin drop to your chest and hold it there for five to ten seconds. Return your head to the neutral position. Slowly let your left ear rest on your left shoulder, again holding it for five to ten seconds. Repeat this with your right side. It is okay if you can't hold your head all the way down. Move until you feel the stretch, but without pain. Do this series three to five times.

■ Shoulder Rounds

Without changing the position of your body, try to exaggerate a shrug upward with your shoulders, bringing them to your ears. Hold this position for five to ten seconds. Then, relax your shoulders back to their beginning position. Move your shoulders in small circles forward for ten repetitions, and then reverse and go backward for ten repetitions.

▓ Wrist/Ankle Rotations

While holding your body in its correct posture, extend your arms in front of you. They should be at your chest level, just below your shoulder. Rotate your wrists forward and backward, about ten small circles each direction. Repeat this exercise with your ankles.

▓ Hip Rotations

This is a lot of fun! Stand with your feet shoulder-width apart and tuck your pelvis in, think of flattening your back. Begin to sway your hips in a clockwise motion, about ten circles. Stop and repeat in a counter-clockwise motion. It looks a lot like belly-dancing!

▓ Calf Stretch

With your hands on your hips and your feet shoulder-width apart, point your toes forward (see **FIGURE 7-3**, p. 100). Step backward with your right foot. The step length should be comfortable and yet a stretch. Ensuring your posture is aligned properly, lean forward, making sure your knee does not extend over your foot (see **FIGURE 7-4**, p. 100). This stretch will be felt in the calf of your rear leg. Do ten of these repetitions and then repeat on the opposite side. If you find yourself in need of some stability while you do this exercise, use a chair placed to one side to hang on to, or even the wall in front of you.

Cooling Down

When you have completed your walk, it is time to cool down. This need not be something extravagant. You can choose to walk at a leisurely pace for the last few minutes of your walk, even if that portion is done in your own driveway. You can even redo your warmup stretches.

Mapping a Course

Where you walk is just as important as the rest of the discussion here. It is best to keep safety in mind at all times. There are many things to consider before going outside for a walk. You will need to pick a time of day to walk that provides you with plenty of time and adequate lighting. Your course should be one that is familiar to you. It should also have sidewalks if at all possible.

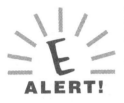

You should alert your family to your walk path, in case they ever needed to find you. Even if you choose several walking paths, be sure to let others know where you are going and when you expect to be home.

Avoid places where there are loose animals. Unless you're up for an unscheduled run, you don't want to be chased by Fido. If the only areas to walk near you include places with animals, try talking to the owners about safety. You might also want to arm yourself with information about local leash laws. Another word on pets, if you choose to walk with your dog, be sure to be kind to your neighbors and clean up after your pet.

Bad Weather Alternatives

When you are in a routine, it is not a lot of fun to have to set that aside simply because of inclement weather. The good thing about walking is that you do not have to be outdoors to do it.

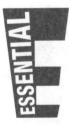

Having a backup plan for the days it is too hot, too cold, or simply yucky outside can save you the headache of coming up with a last-minute idea of where to walk. Look around your neighbor-hood and see where other walkers go during inclement weather. Follow the masses!

Mall Walking

If you live near a mall, there are probably a good number of walkers who frequent the mall. Many malls offer special hours to mall walkers, usually prior to the opening of the stores. Sometimes it's even after the stores close. Many mall walkers prefer to go before the crowds arrive.

You can simply call the mall offices to ask about mall walking rules and hours. They can also give you an idea of the distances and courses in the mall. Most of the time, they have already been mapped out for you. Some malls even offer special discounts to their walkers. So even if you don't use the mall often, there may be some perks for you to sign up as a mall walker.

The benefits of mall walking are usually that it is free, convenient, and safe. Many malls have security guards located on premises twenty-four hours a day. The parking lots are well lit if you use their facilities after-hours or during hours when it may be dark and deserted. Another benefit is that you're not walking alone. Even if you don't set out to walk with a group, many people who start walking at the mall often find they fall into a group quite easily. The mall is also a great place to walk with a new baby, because of the constant temperature.

Fitness Facilities

Fitness clubs or facilities are also another place where you can walk should the weather or timing be a problem for your walking. Many have tracks around the center that are mapped out for you, mileage wise. You may have to share this track with some joggers.

ALERT!

Be sure to ask about the hours of operation, the fees involved, and the commitments. Some facilities will even let you have a trial membership to see if their services are what you need. However, you should be very careful before signing anything. Read the fine print first!

Benefits to the use of a fitness facility or gym include locker rooms and showers, appropriate flooring, access to mentors or personal trainers, and many others. Unfortunately, many facilities charge you for these extra features. This cost is usually charged whether you use their gym or not. If you like having the added facility and do not mind the extra cost, this might be the right option for you. You would definitely have other benefits besides simply the walking track, including other classes, meeting other members, and added options for exercise.

Treadmills

So it is raining outside and you can't walk. You don't have the option of a mall or fitness facility. What is left for you to do? Some women choose to purchase a treadmill for general use or for use on days when it is rainy. This can be a great option. Although there is a cost commitment, it is yours forever, unlike a gym membership. You can also share its use with your spouse or others in your home.

Stairs

Say a treadmill isn't for you? Consider using your stairs. This can actually be a great workout. Remember to watch your balance and your levels of exertion. Just because you are not at the gym or outside, doesn't mean you can't overdo it.

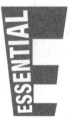

If you choose to walk outside in inclement weather, be sure to take necessary precautions. You will want to wear bright, reflective clothing, and carry a cell phone in case you need to be picked up. Also bring along an umbrella or other protective gear for your walk. Remember that cars can't see you very well in poor lighting conditions or bad weather, so be wise when you walk.

Walking Benefits in Pregnancy

Walking is beneficial to you in many ways. It provides you with an appropriate form of aerobic exercise. Yet it is low impact and easy to do. While your body is changing, walking does not require a great deal of skill or balance. Chances are you probably know how to walk already. You can adapt walking to be as strenuous as you require your exercise to be. It is also gentle enough that even if you have never exercised you can begin to do it in pregnancy. (E)

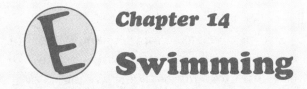

Chapter 14

Swimming

Swimming is probably one of the best exercises a pregnant woman can do. Not only is it a great workout, but also the buoyancy of the water can help alleviate many problems (such as overheating and jarring movements) associated with exercise and pregnancy. Pregnant women also report feeling great being in the water.

The Surprising Benefits of Swimming

When you think of swimming, you might remember lazy days splashing around the pool as a child. Or if you already have children, the thought of the pool might even have the negative connotations of getting everyone together, fighting the crowds, and baking in the sun. While both of these may be accurate representations of swimming, they don't have much to do with swimming while pregnant.

Swimming is a favorite form of exercise for pregnant women for a variety of reasons. It provides you with a great cardiovascular workout and exercises the majority of your muscle groups. Many women enjoy the feeling of floating and taking stress off their bones and joints. Others enjoy the cool feelings they have while in the pool, even during the colder months. Some just find the water relaxing.

Overall, swimming is an excellent way to stay physically and mentally fit during your pregnancy. Swimming also offers the added benefit of being readily available to all fitness levels.

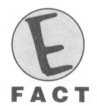

FACT

When you are in water, you feel much lighter than on the land. For example, 150 pounds feels like it weighs about 15 pounds while submerged. This feels great when you're sporting the extra pounds of pregnancy!

Open to All

Swimming is one of the few exercises that you can do during pregnancy, even if you have not been a frequent exerciser prior to pregnancy. This is good news for you if you've not previously been swimming, or if your overall fitness level is not as high as you'd like it to be. You can start by swimming easily for twenty minutes a day. Do this three to four times a week.

Movement

Being pregnant can cause a variety of weight-related problems, particularly when it comes to your joints and bones. While in water, you feel lighter and do not have as many concerns with the bumping and jarring of being on land. The more pregnant you become, the more relaxin (a hormone secreted by the placenta and the lining of the uterus) your body releases. While this is of great benefit during labor, when you want your pelvis to move more freely, it can cause a variety of aches and pains during pregnancy.

The buoyancy of the water allows you to move around freely. Many pregnant women report feeling lighter and more limber while in water. This beneficial aspect can help make your workout easier, not to mention its effect on pain relief! Buoyancy also helps protect you from injury due to exercise.

Posture Aid

Being in the pool also aids with your posture. It's easier to be upright in the pool. Maintaining proper positioning of your body will help alleviate and prevent some problems associated with pregnancy. The water also acts as a massage agent by exerting force on your body and massaging your muscles as you move around.

Being in the water does require some balance. This is something you may struggle with during pregnancy. However, in the water you're not as likely to fall and injure yourself as you may be on land. This adds difficulty to the workout while still allowing you to exercise your balance and work on improvements.

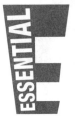

You can also use the buoyancy of the water to provide resistance for your workouts. Using the water to ease your workouts and increase the difficulty can take some time, so just get used to the feel of the water first, if you're not used to exercising in the aquatic environment.

Relaxation

Just as when you were a kid, swimming or even being in water can leave you physically exhausted. While you may feel exhausted on a general basis, this form of exhaustion and relaxation is more conducive to sleeping than general pregnancy exhaustion.

We know that exercising helps pregnant women and others get more rest at night. Exercising in water has this same benefit. In addition, exercise in water offers the added benefit of feeling less weighed down by the added weight of pregnancy; others are simply more relaxed in water.

Blood Pressure

Ah, here's a great benefit that many people do not know about. If you have blood pressure problems, particularly while pregnant, simply being in shoulder-deep water can help decrease your overall blood pressure. This is due to increased circulation and relief from swelling. There is also a decrease in the associated risks of high blood pressure.

Breech Babies

Some studies indicate that you can use a pool and water to help turn a breech baby, or a baby that is not in a head-down position. The methods to do this are varied. One involves the pregnant woman doing handstands in water that comes up to the top of her thighs. The other is having her dive into the pool. Apparently, these exercises are supposed to help turn a breech baby. However, always check with your doctor or midwife before doing these types of exercises.

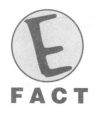

FACT

Beginning at about twenty-eight weeks of gestation, babies will start to move into a head-down position. Babies are breech about 3 to 4 percent of the time at your due date. If your baby is still breech at your due date or before, you can try exercises and even external version (manually turning baby, done by your practitioner) to turn the baby head down. If these attempts are unsuccessful, most practitioners recommend a cesarean birth.

Water Aerobics

Water aerobics is great fun! Many gyms and fitness centers now offer water aerobics as a part of their programs. Some even specifically have pregnancy water aerobics. While it is not necessary to find a class that is specifically geared toward pregnancy, it is imperative that you talk to the instructor about your pregnancy. This allows him or her to alert you to changes you need to make while participating in the class.

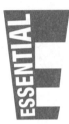

Scuba diving is never recommended in pregnancy. This holds true even if you're an experienced diver. There is simply too much danger involved for the baby. Switch to snorkeling in the pool until you've had your baby.

Precautions

Exercising in water can be very deceptive—you get a great workout with what feels like less effort. It is also possible to be overheated, even though you're in water. If you feel dizzy or lightheaded, tell the instructor or someone near you and get help to the edge of the pool or out of the pool.

Here are also a few reasons why exercise in water would not be appropriate:

- If your amniotic sac, or bag of waters, was broken or leaking
- If you had an infection
- If you were experiencing preterm labor or another contraindication to exercise

Simple Exercises for the Pool

Not everyone will be able to find or attend an organized swimming class or water aerobics session. This doesn't mean that you can't benefit from water aerobics as a form of pregnancy exercise. Simply find your own workout for the pool.

Pool Walking

By breathing naturally, and walking around the pool as you would on the ground, you can get some good exercise. This is called "traveling in the pool." You can do other exercises and then spend a few minutes walking around the pool. Over the course of your workout you will accumulate this traveling time into a workout of its own. This is best done in shallow water, no higher than waist deep.

Pool Jogging

Unlike regular jogging, which can be jarring to the system, running in water offers you some padding. It is often used to help runners rehabilitate after an injury, or surgery, as an acceptable form of running. So, if running and pregnancy sound good to you, but don't seem to go together, try running in the pool.

The basics are the same as for running outside the pool. You can even wear your running shoes, though they are not necessary. You can run in place or move around in a small area of the pool.

For an added workout, add your arms while you run. If this is too much work, you can always stop the arm movements. Remember to warm up and cool down, even in the pool.

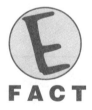

FACT

Just moving in the water takes more energy than moving outside the pool. The resistance from the water is what helps provide you with the workout. So if you find yourself in the pool, just move around and see how you start to feel. With a bit of coordination, it's a complete workout!

Hanging on to the Edge

The edge of the pool is a great place to work out. This is particularly true if you're concerned about floating away, or if you're not incredibly tall.

Go to the edge of the pool and hang on to the lip of the pool. Be sure to avoid the areas where there are drains or stairs. These will be more dangerous and high traffic areas.

Hang on and just start moving. It doesn't matter if you face in or out. Try some simple flutters with your feet. You can advance to more full-fledged kicking as you feel you are able to do so. This will provide you with a safe and quiet workout without leaving the pool.

Treading Water

Treading water also falls into this category. While you might believe it to be just child's play or something done to prove you won't drown yourself, treading water is a great workout. The movement of your arms and legs will keep you afloat but also provide you with a lot of exercise for two large muscle groups.

Your legs aren't what you want to move? Try doing some basic arm movements, like circles. Alternate big circles with small circles. Go forward and backward in direction. Hold your arms in front of your chest with your arms bent in and twist slowly at the waist.

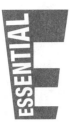

Chlorine exposure is minimal while swimming, but for added safety and to decrease potential exposure, always end your workout session with a shower to rinse off any chemicals from the pool. This is good advice for any swimmer.

Even bouncing up and down while making splashing movements with your arms can be fun and a good workout. For some added workout, try to propel yourself out of the pool, like a rocket. First, bend your knees slightly and then push up with your feet while you push down with your arms. Even kids can get into this exercise.

Lower Body Workout

■ Squatting

Go to the water level that is chest deep for you. Place your feet about hip-width apart and keep your toes pointing forward. Sit back with your bottom and allow your arms to come up to the front, chest level for balance. Push yourself back to the original pose using your feet, while bringing your arms to the sides. This can be a very easy exercise. To make it harder, try doing it in shallower water. Remember, squats help prepare your body for birth. The repetitive strengthening of the leg muscles helps you assume positions of birth to make it faster and easier for you. Try this exercise for eight to ten repetitions.

■ Lunges

In chest-deep water, stand again with your feet hip-width apart. Take a step backward, placing your weight between the sole of the front foot and the ball of your back foot. Bend your knees until you've reached as far as you can go. You should not go lower than is comfortable or so low that your neck is underwater. Hold the pose for a few seconds and then push up to your original pose. You can alternate feet or do one side at a time. You should do eight to ten repetitions of this exercise for full benefit. Again, to increase the difficulty of this exercise, try doing it in shallower water.

■ Leg Lifts

This is another simple exercise you can do while in the pool. In chest-deep water, stand with your feet hip-width apart. Stand with soft knees and bring your left leg up toward the surface, toes pointed up. Go as far as you can without losing balance or injuring yourself. Repeat this eight to ten times and then switch legs.

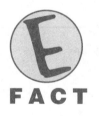

FACT

Water temperature is still important in pregnancy. Most pools keep their water temperature between 82 and 86 degrees Fahrenheit. This temperature level is fine for pregnant women. Be sure to see where the water temperature of your pool is posted and check it daily.

Exercise Aids

While swimming or doing water aerobics, some pregnant women desire using some of the varied exercise aids. These can include water weights, flotation devices, and so forth.

You might consider using them to help you exercise or to help you relax. Many moms resort to using flotation devices in the final months of pregnancy. This allows more of your body to remain underwater, while allowing you to float, much like your baby floats.

Kick boards are another water aid that can be useful while pregnant. Try taking a kick board with you as you semi-float around the pool. It can be useful to lie your head on as you float, or you can use it to hang on to while kicking your legs away.

A deep-water flotation belt can be handy if you aren't the best swimmer or you are trying to do your workouts in the deep end. The problem is that by the end of the second trimester, the belt may not fit your growing abdomen. Exercise caution when in deep water and talk to the lifeguards and other pool personnel about the use of flotation belts.

The Lap Lane

For the experienced swimmer, the lap lane is the place where it all happens. You get your lane and you go. This can be a very wonderful form of exercise. It allows you to set the pace and control how far you go. As you progress in pregnancy, you may find that you have no trouble maintaining your normal lap schedule. If you do need to cut back either in distance or speed, it's easily adjusted.

ESSENTIAL

When swimming, be sure to watch your form. Kicking too vigorously has the potential to injure your pubic symphysis because of the added hormone relaxin. Flutter kicking is fine, as is moderate breaststroke kicking, just don't overdo it.

Be sure you know the rules of your lap pool. Is there a certain way to turn around? If it involves going underwater, are you okay with that? What about which direction you swim in? Some pools have alternating directions. Will you be expected to share lanes? Is there a time limit to how long you can have a lane? Be sure you know these rules of the pool before you jump in.

Where to Swim

Finding the time to exercise is always talked about, but what about finding a place to swim? Many people are lucky enough to have indoor pools located fairly close to their homes. And the majority of us know where to swim in the summer. However, choosing a place to swim for exercise might be a completely different task than swimming with the kids.

You will want to find a place that has not only convenient hours and locations, but also fees that are reasonable. Many locations offer swim-only memberships. Some natatoriums offer discounts if you take their classes. Be sure to check out the prices and availability. Nothing is more frustrating than going to swim to find the lap lanes filled with a toddler class.

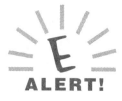

ALERT!

Watch being out in the sun during pregnancy. Your skin is more sensitive. You might be more likely to burn or develop splotches from exposure. Sunscreen will help you protect your pregnant glow without the fear of the splotchy skin.

Check your local YMCA, JCC, and even local colleges for places to swim indoors. Many outdoor pools are also joining the competition and placing bubbles, heated covers, and plastic buildings over their pools to make them accessible in the winter. You might even ask members of local swim clubs for their recommendations for wintertime swimming locations. Ⓔ

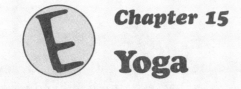

Chapter 15

Yoga

The use of yoga during pregnancy may be the perfect combination of exercise, centering, and relaxation. Not only will this exercise form work out your body, but it will allow you to exercise your mind and help relieve stress as well. It is also easily adapted for all fitness levels, including some women on bed rest or women with exercise restrictions during pregnancy.

What Is Yoga?

Yoga is derived from the Sanskrit word *yuk*, which means "yoke," or to join together. The basic translation has come to be "union." Using the concept of the union of body, mind, and soul, yoga offers many benefits to you during your pregnancy, birth, and postpartum. Some practitioners look at it as a bonding of mother and baby, even before birth.

Yoga Benefits

The benefits of yoga go beyond the typical benefits of the physical body. Yoga is definitely a fitness activity that takes the mind and soul into consideration as well. This can be very useful to you as you begin your journey into parenthood, even if it is not the first time you have been down this path.

Yoga is actually a generic term used to encompass many different forms of yoga. Hatha yoga, iyengar yoga, and ashtanga yoga are the most common forms in the Western world. But there are many more forms of yoga. Each of these forms employs an ancient concept of physical well-being and balance with the mental and spiritual side of your body and soul. They stress strength, relaxation, and flexibility as a way to unite the body.

By using poses or *asanas*, you learn to strengthen your body. You increase your flexibility. You develop a sense of inner wisdom as you learn more about your pregnant body.

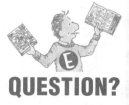

QUESTION?

What should I wear for yoga?
You can wear anything that is comfortable to you. Most practitioners recommend loose enough clothing that you are relaxed and not irritated, but not so loose as to get in the way of your poses or balance. It is best to do yoga while not wearing shoes or socks. If you choose form-fitted clothing, be sure it allows your skin to breathe.

Yoga as a Process

It is also important to note that yoga is process-oriented rather than goal-oriented. This means it does not matter how many times you perform a movement or pose, but that you focus on it while participating fully. Tackle each pose as if it is the only pose you will do. Focus completely and entirely on the pose as you do it. Do not let your mind wander to the next pose or the day ahead. This is a different viewpoint from regular exercise that frequently focuses on the number of repetitions.

Stress Reduction

Stress is something that has a negative effect on our lives. For the most part, we have more than enough stress to deal with. Yoga has been used for centuries to help reduce the amount of stress felt by an individual. Pregnancy creates stressors that you may not anticipate, even if this is a much-planned pregnancy. Yoga accomplishes this stress reduction with a few simple techniques: centering, breathing, and poses.

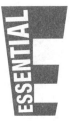

When you do your yoga is as important as *how* you do it. Most instructors recommend that if you can make it happen, doing yoga before breakfast is optimal. It is said your mind is calmer than after a hectic day of typical stressors. Experiment with the times of day you do your workout and see what works best for you.

Centering

This is another way of saying get in touch with your body. Through a combination of breathing, poses, and centering, you will learn techniques to help you and your body through pregnancy. Often this component of yoga is referred to as meditation.

Meditation requires practice and skill. It is not something that comes automatically to many people. During pregnancy, learning the ability to put other thoughts out of your mind and to focus on your body and your baby will have many benefits.

The Breathing

Say the word *breathing* to nearly any pregnant woman and her mind immediately goes to the old patterned paced breathing, often associated with panting dogs and laboring women. Not only is this form of breathing not appropriate for labor and birth, it's not great for pregnant women either. Breathing in yoga is a completely different form.

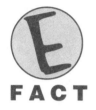

FACT

Breathing is a known way to reduce stress and to increase relaxation. This is the foundation of most childbirth classes. What type of breathing is practiced varies from organization to organization. Be sure to ask your potential teachers which form of breathing they use.

The Yoga Breath

Ujayi breathing, or the yoga breath, is said to promote calmness and a feeling of well-being. During your pregnancy, practicing this form of breathing can be beneficial to you and your baby in many ways. It will help you learn relaxation techniques that are beneficial for labor. As your mind and body relax, you are better able to give birth with reduced amounts of pain.

To learn this technique, you will need to practice. Slowly intake your breath, filling your belly or abdomen first, and then draw the air up into your lungs until they fill and your rib cage separates. Then slowly exhale all of the air until your lungs are completely empty. You can add thoughts to the breathing as well.

For example, imagine, as you breathe in that you are bringing good, clean air to your baby. "See" that breath travel down through your body and through the placenta and umbilical cord to your baby. Then as you exhale, imagine carrying away all the toxins in your body, away from your baby.

Breath Control

Learning to control your breath is also important in the pushing phase of labor. Doing yoga-type breathing during this phase will increase your oxygen levels as well as those of your baby. This makes it safer and more satisfying for you as you push your baby into this world.

ALERT!

Holding your breath in labor while pushing can decrease the amounts of oxygen to you and your baby. It can also lead to excessive straining, which can cause hemorrhoids or even tearing of the perineum if the baby is born too quickly.

Poses

There are many poses involved in yoga. Many of these poses are perfectly appropriate for pregnancy. Using them alone or in conjunction with other forms of exercise can greatly enhance your skills and preparation.

Remember when doing poses, never do them to the point of exhaustion. Never bend or stretch further than is comfortable. And hold them only as long as you feel steady and relaxed.

Sample Yoga Poses

■ Child's Pose

Kneel on the floor, separating your knees slightly. Put your big toes together and sit back with your buttocks on the heels of your feet. Stretch your arms over your head (see **FIGURE 5-12**, p. 63). Hold this pose for five seconds, releasing a bit more with each breath. If this reach is too far for you as a beginner or later in pregnancy, bend your elbows and rest on your forearms to alleviate some of the tension.

■ Forward Bend

Stand with your feet as wide apart as comfortable. Lean forward onto two supports to hold your body weight. Focus on keeping your chest open. Hold your head up to allow a good stretch of your neck (see **FIGURE 15-1**).

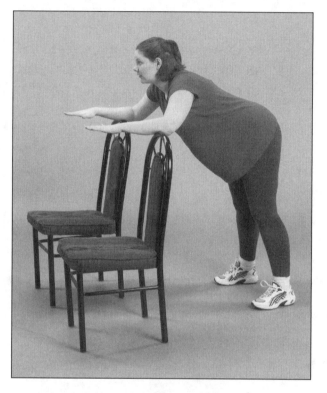

FIGURE 15-1
Forward Bend—Enjoy the stretch of the chest and upper back

■ Modified Forward Bend

To open the pelvic area, sit on floor, with your thighs spread apart to accommodate your growing abdomen. Bend forward at the back and hold your toes with your hands if you can. Keep the knees straight.

■ Cat Balance

While kneeling on the floor, pull in your abdominal muscles and breathe naturally. As you exhale, extend your right leg and left arm. Think about extending each limb as far as you comfortably can. Hold this pose for three to five breaths. Repeat ten times on each side.

■ Modified Cobra Pose

Stand with feet together, or separated if that is more comfortable, with your hands clasped behind your back. Inhale and drop your head back. Hold this pose and breathe gently (see **FIGURE 15-2**). Inhale again arching your back, while pushing your chest out and your arms back. Finally, push your hips forward. This can avoid abdominal pressure and strengthen the legs while giving your back a good stretch and backward bend.

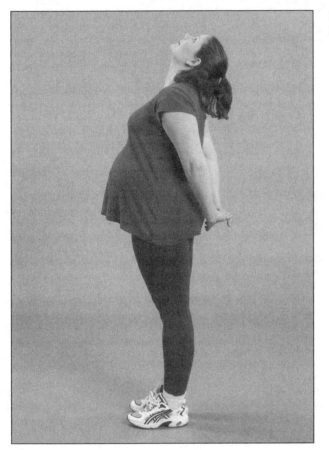

FIGURE 15-2
Modified Cobra Pose

■ Wall Butterfly

Lie down on the floor with your bottom and feet against the wall, keep your soles together, and let your knees drop open. Use your hands to press your knees downward toward the wall (see **FIGURE 15-3**). This exercise will open up your pelvic area. It also helps to strengthen your legs, inner thighs, and lower spine.

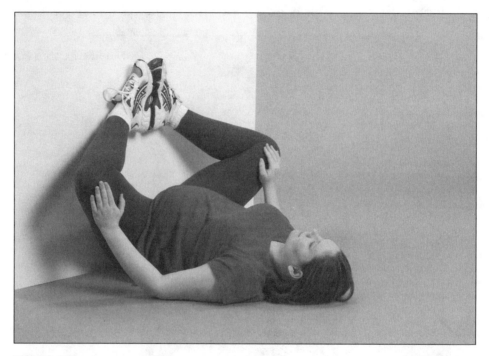

FIGURE 15-3
Wall Butterfly

You can also do this pose seated with a partner. Simply sit and pull your knees up as close as comfortable to your body. Have your partner hold your outer legs at about knee level. Have him or her provide slight resistance as you try to separate your legs. This is a great way to get others involved in your pregnancy! Even a school-aged child can help here.

■ Wall Squat

Standing up straight with your back facing a wall, place the birth ball between you and the wall around the center of your back and press it into the wall using your back. Slowly walk your feet forward, leaning back into the ball for support (see **FIGURE 7-6**, p. 102). As you walk forward, the ball will roll up to the center of your back, between your shoulder blades. This allows you to do a squat without having to worry about being steady or having a partner (see **FIGURE 7-7**, p. 102). When you are down as far as you can go, hold the pose for up to ten seconds, and then slowly walk your feet back to their starting position, allowing the ball to roll back to the center of your lower back.

■ Down Dog

This is not a beginner pose. Stand with your feet hip-width apart. Bend at the hips over a collection of supports or a chair. This can be a stack of towels or blankets over a bed, or anything about waist height. Rest your hands and your arms on the supports in front of you (see **FIGURE 15-4**). Your head will probably be about thigh level, depending on your flexibility. If your heels come up off the floor, have someone place supports under your feet. You may require help getting into this pose.

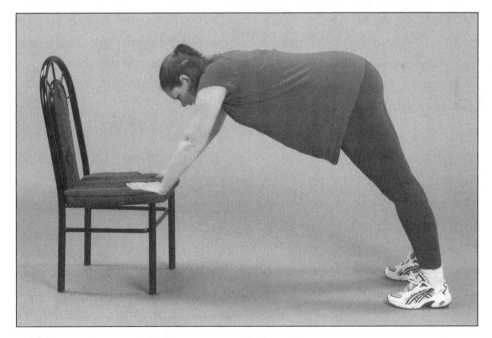

FIGURE 15-4
Down Dog Pose

Using these techniques to help you achieve a physical, mental, and emotional balance is very easy to do. You should aim to do yoga about fifteen minutes a day, a couple of days a week, with the remainder of the days doing twenty to thirty minutes of yoga. This will provide you a good balance.

Yoga Practice Choices

Yoga does not have to be done in a classroom, nor does it have to be done alone. There are a variety of ways to approach your yoga education.

Yoga Classes

There are plenty of yoga classes available in most cities. There are also more and more classes for pregnancy yoga. To find out what is available where you live, try looking up yoga in the phone book and calling some different centers.

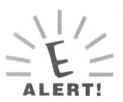

ALERT!

While other exercise classes offer teachers with certification, there is no such thing as a national or international certification for a yoga instructor. This is partially because there are many forms of yoga and many different organizations. Look for an instructor with a long history of teaching. Ask to speak to other students in the class for their opinion.

If they do offer yoga classes specifically for pregnancy, ask about the class population. Is it made up of beginners? Or are a variety of levels taught in one class? Does the instructor have any specific pregnancy-related credentials?

Classes are nice because they offer a built-in support system and an instructor to help you answer questions and make suggestions. If the class is comprised of other pregnant women, it can really be helpful that you are all experiencing similar life changes. But classes are not necessary for the success of your yoga program.

Yoga Videos

Yoga videos can be another great way to experience yoga during pregnancy. There are many forms of yoga classes available on tape from a wide variety of instructors. Always try to get a reference for a good video from a yoga practitioner or even reviews of tapes. This can prevent you from going through several tapes trying to find the right fit.

Yoga Books

There are also many yoga books with sections on pregnancy and yoga. There are also quite a few yoga books specifically designed for pregnant women. Look for books with clear instructions and photos to help you. Also ask around to see what books others are using.

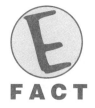

FACT

When doing yoga on your own, make sure you choose a well-ventilated room for your practice sessions. Level flooring is also important to your balance issues. Bring any props you will need, such as a mat, strap, or blanket. The room should be free of distractions, drafts, and moisture.

Yoga Precautions

Although yoga is a great form of exercise for pregnancy, there are a few precautions you must remember. The first thing to remember is that above all else, if anything hurts—stop. This is a basic rule of exercise during pregnancy. You may tend to forget about yoga as a form of exercise, but these basics still hold true.

Pregnancy is an acceptable time to start yoga, even if you have never done it before. Some instructors advise that you wait until you are in the second trimester to begin yoga if you have never done it before. However, in absence of any medical indications not to exercise, yoga is perfectly acceptable in the first trimester. Always let your instructor know you are expecting.

Remember that your body is full of hormones, including relaxin. This will cause you to be more susceptible to injury, including overstretching. Listen to your body. It will provide you with signals that you are going too far. Use towels and bands to help you reach your feet in certain poses.

When bending, remember to bend at the back, not at your hips. This will be more comfortable on your body. Keeping your upper back as straight as possible will also help decrease discomfort and breathing difficulties. In a seated position, use the towel around your feet to help remain upright.

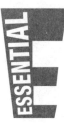

Remember to give your baby room as you are doing poses. If you need to modify a pose to fit your expanding abdomen, simply try spreading your legs a bit wider, although you do need to focus on balance as well.

Balance Issues

Many poses in yoga will require balance. This is something you don't have a lot of while pregnant. Try to do these poses near the wall or a chair to help you maintain your balance, particularly after the fourth month. If this is not possible, skip these poses and save them for postpartum use.

Poses that require you to lie on your back or stomach should be avoided after about four months of pregnancy. If you find they are uncomfortable sooner, discontinue them at that point. Don't wait until a certain arbitrary time. Always use good judgment while doing any form of exercise. Remember, listen to your body.

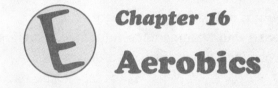

Chapter 16

Aerobics

The aerobics craze has hit pregnancy! If you like a rise in your heart rate, this might be for you. If you have been doing aerobics for years, continuing with it might be the natural progression for your pregnancy. Many people find themselves addicted to this type of workout. Learn how to play it safe, smart, and healthy while doing aerobics during your pregnancy.

THE EVERYTHING PREGNANCY FITNESS BOOK

Aerobic Benefits in Pregnancy

Aerobics literally means "with oxygen." This means that aerobics is a form of exercise that requires additional oxygen and so, in response to this need, your lungs and heart work harder to provide the extra oxygen that is required. As your heart and lungs are muscles, aerobics also provides them with an additional workout. By working out your heart and lungs during pregnancy, you not only strengthen the muscular components, but also increase your stamina and endurance, which is of great benefit during your pregnancy, labor, birth, and beyond.

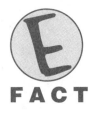

FACT

Aerobic exercise in pregnancy can help lower your blood pressure. During the actual exercise your blood pressure may rise, but overall the conditioning and toning from the exercise will allow your body to have a lowered blood pressure.

Aerobics in Your Daily Life

Aerobic exercise probably calls to mind skinny women dressed in leotards, dancing at a rapid pace to loud rock music. While this is certainly one form of aerobic exercise, there are many others. In fact, you probably get more aerobic exercise than you might think.

All of the walking, running, and swimming that you do requires the use of oxygen and is, therefore, aerobic. However, without intending to use these as your form of exercise, it can be hard to get the workout your body really needs. If you specifically set out to use your daily activities as a form of exercise, it only takes a bit of thought to make that happen.

How could you incorporate a walk into your daily routine? You could begin to walk to work. Perhaps you could bicycle your toddler to preschool? What about everyday errands? Could you walk to the grocery store to pick up ingredients for dinner? What if you need to send a package from the office overnight, can you walk to the postal service center?

Safety Measures

You may be one of the many women who already does aerobics as her personal form of exercise. If so, you may already be accustomed to the rigors of aerobics. However, during your pregnancy, there are certain precautions to be taken, as with any form of exercise in pregnancy. For aerobics during pregnancy, most of them revolve around your heart rate, your core body temperature, and your exertion levels.

Heart Rate

Heart rate issues in pregnant women are commonly heard about. The reason that heart rate is used is that it is an indirect prediction of how much oxygen is being used. The one problem is finding the one heart rate number that works for you. The most often quoted heart rate that is appropriate during pregnancy exercise will be 140 beats per minute (bpm).

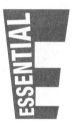

When taking your pulse, always be sure that you do not completely restrict blood flow through the artery that you are using. It is also not a good idea to use the carotid artery (in your neck) to take your pulse. Use an artery in your wrist or elsewhere when taking your pulse during pregnancy.

Your aerobics class instructor should allot at least one, but preferably two, periods of time to check your heart rate during class. These can easily be incorporated into the workout. If your instructor doesn't incorporate them into class, or only does one official period, never hesitate to slow it down and take your pulse yourself.

It is also important that you know your resting heart rate. Remember that during pregnancy your resting heart rate will probably be a bit higher. Again, this is due to the added blood volume needed to sustain your pregnancy. To obtain your resting heart rate, simply take your pulse in the morning before getting out of bed. Try doing this several mornings in a row for a better average.

A heart rate of 140 beats per minute will be good if you are not used to working out often. It is also beneficial if you do not regularly follow your target heart rate closely while exercising. It winds up being a very nice goal if you are in one of these situations. However, if you are used to exercising a lot, 140 beats per minute is not a great workout for you at all. You may find that if you are very athletic, 140 beats per minute is very easily attained and maintained without much exertion on your part. This can prevent you from making the most of your workout. It is best to consult your trainer, health-care provider, and other people involved in your physical fitness quests. Sometimes there is simply not a "one size fits all" approach to heart rate.

Body Temperature Issues

The first trimester is when your baby is most vulnerable to development problems. These potential problems can come from many factors, including what you eat, drink, or inhale. Many women don't realize that body temperature issues, like a hot tub, hot bath or shower, fevers, and extremes in elevated body temperature can also cause problems.

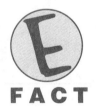

According to the American College of Obstetrics and Gynecology (ACOG), your body temperature should not be above 101 degrees Fahrenheit axillary (under your arm) after exercising. If it is, you've done too much and need to re-evaluate your program.

Your core body temperature is also very important, particularly in the first trimester of pregnancy. During the first trimester, an elevated core body temperature can be raised to the point that damage can be done to your growing baby. Though we often talk about this happening, it is not very commonly done. By addressing health concerns quickly, avoiding hot tubs, baths, and showers, and generally avoiding overheating, you can prevent this from affecting your baby.

Dehydration can cause your body temperature to rise. Always drink plenty of water when you exercise—before, during, and after your workout.

You need to drink water continuously. You should plan on consuming at least 16 ounces of water during the two-hour period before you intend to work out, according to new guidelines set forth by the American College of Sports Medicine. They also recommend 5 to 12 ounces for every fifteen to twenty minutes that you're actually working out. Follow up your workout by drinking 16 ounces of water.

Workout Environment

The place in which you work out is also a source of potential problems. If the room is too warm, you will find yourself becoming too warm very quickly. Remember, you've got an expanded blood volume that makes becoming overheated fairly simple. Ensure that the room is of an adequate temperature and has ventilation.

Your clothing also plays a part in your ability to heat or cool your body. Wearing layers that can be removed during your workout is a great idea. After your warmup, simply remove your top layer and proceed with your exercise routine.

If you choose to exercise outdoors, watch the thermometer. Avoid being outside for prolonged periods in extreme weather. It's very easy to overheat in the summer months, even following clothing and water precautions.

ALERT!

During the third trimester of pregnancy, as your blood volume expands more and the number of times you breathe per minute goes up, it becomes much easier to raise your heart rate. Be sure to plan for this while you exercise during the third trimester. Slowing it down is the best way to reduce your heart rate.

Exertion Level

Exertion levels are another core element in determining if you are doing too much when you work out. As we've talked about before, the talk test is a good idea to keep in mind. Can you talk to the person next to you without gasping for air? If not, slow it down!

One of the easiest ways to slow your workout down in aerobics is to not combine large muscle groups during exercise. For example, do your arm work but not your leg work or vice versa. You can do them separately, just not all at once.

Class Modification Options

Nearly any form of aerobics is safe during your pregnancy. Though it's always best to stick to familiar but modified routines. It is also wise to avoid high-impact aerobics. If you are currently involved in a class that is doing aerobics, be sure to tell the instructor you're expecting. If they have prenatal aerobics classes, you might consider moving to those; if not, ask the instructor what you can do to modify the current class.

If the intensity of your workout becomes too much for you to handle, you can always quickly decrease it. To do this, simply drop the arm movements from whatever you are doing or decrease the pace or number of the repetitions of that particular exercise. You may find that certain exercises routinely cause you to feel overworked, while others don't bother you. This is probably due to your fitness level or skill set prior to this pregnancy. This is a very easy way to keep your workout going, without injuring you or your baby.

ESSENTIAL

Maintaining your balance can be a big problem during pregnancy, particularly as your center of gravity changes during the fourth month onward. As you do an aerobics routine, you can easily get off balance. Try doing your routine near a chair or wall that you can hang on to for support.

Evaluating a Prenatal Class and Instructor

If you are lucky enough to have found an actual prenatal aerobics class and a prenatal fitness instructor, you might want to watch or take a sample class before signing up. As with anything in life, not all things are equal.

You may find that the class does not fit your pregnancy needs. Here are some questions to ask your instructor or observe about the class:

- Do the times of the class fit your schedule?
- What is the missed class policy?
- How is the class modified for pregnancy?
- At what point do they allow you in the class?
- Are postpartum women in the class as well? If so, does the class do something different for them?

You will also want to check your instructor's credentials. What type of pregnancy training does he or she have? Does he or she hold any special certifications? What philosophy does he or she have about pregnancy and exercise? These types of questions will help fill you in on how much practical experience and knowledge the instructor has about the differences pregnancy creates for the prenatal aerobics class.

Talk to Class Members

Be sure to talk to other members of the aerobics class before you join. Find out what type of fitness level backgrounds they had prior to pregnancy and how they feel they are doing in the class. Ask about alumni of the class. If postpartum women aren't included, does the location offer postpartum classes? Or are you expected to go into a regular aerobics class after you give birth to your baby?

Get Workout Videos

Even if you can't find a class that meets your pregnancy or postpartum needs in your area, there are other ways to get your aerobics in. There are many videos on the subject from a variety of standpoints. Perhaps you're used to doing aerobics via video. If you have an instructor or series that you like, chances are he or she makes a pregnancy version. Videotapes can be a really good alternative, particularly since you'll know the instructor's style and habits. This can make the transition go more smoothly.

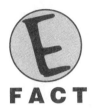

Some videos are taught by instructors who are pregnant themselves. Using a video that offers other pregnant women as the models is beneficial. It can show you the variety of stages of growth and how different bellies can look from woman to woman.

Some videos also offer the postpartum workout. This is a nice touch for a complete series of workouts. It will help address specific postpartum needs and is usually done in a rather efficient manner because, as a new mom, you probably don't have a lot of extra time to spare. Also look at a video series and ask who are the women in this segment of the video? Again, continuity will win out in my book. Do the same women come back to exercise with you?

Aerobic Exercises for Pregnancy

While you might think of aerobics as being one certain set of exercises, it is certainly not true. Here you will not find a list of exactly what to do to get a great workout for your pregnant body, but rather some ideas of getting aerobic exercise on a regular basis, whether from a prenatal aerobics class or on your own. The key to aerobics is to remember that you need to do it three to four times a week, for twenty to thirty minutes each time.

Bicycling

Bicycling can be a great form of exercise during pregnancy. Though some practitioners will tell you to park your bike around twenty to twenty-four weeks for balance issues. They do agree that stationary bikes can be used until you give birth to your baby.

Whether you ride your regular bike or a stationary bike, the aerobics workout you'll get is great. If you're riding your real bike, you also have the options of taking children along in bike seats, going with friends or your partner, or simply getting out and enjoying the neighborhood on your own. Be sure always to wear your helmet and to carry water in water bottles to prevent dehydration.

Stationary bikes offer the advantage of not requiring helmets and of always being indoors. This prevents you from getting soaked or having to worry about traffic and other outdoor concerns. Some bikes will come with several riding "programs" that you choose. Find a program that works well for you without being too tiring. If the bike isn't a programmable one, you might consider a cycling class offered through many fitness centers. Your other option is to ride as you wish on the bike.

May I still do step aerobics?
The answer is a resounding yes! Step aerobics is a great form of exercise for you during pregnancy, particularly if it's something your body is used to doing. Other than balance concerns and modifying the workout to include slower changes in direction, you should be fine.

QUESTION?

Fitness Machines

There are also a wealth of fitness machines available in fitness centers. Or you might actually own one yourself. Either way, these are also great ways to fit aerobics into your exercise habit. The only ones you should really avoid during pregnancy are those that use a sliding motion. With your balance being off and the odd positions required, it is more likely to hurt you than provide you with a good pregnancy workout.

Stair steppers, elliptical machines, treadmills, ski machines, and the like are all perfect workout opportunities for you during your pregnancy. It may be easier for you to use a lowered setting or program, particularly if you are not used to using the machines. You can also just do it freestyle to find what meets your needs on any given day.

Warmup Aerobics

As with all exercise you can't neglect the warmup. In aerobics, the warmup is meant to help prepare you for the workout. It tends to include stretching and movement of the major muscle groups.

■ Marching

Stand with your feet slightly apart and your arms loosely at your side. Begin by marching, or exaggerated walking, by bringing your knees up one at a time and returning them to the floor, alternating feet. You should take care not to stomp your feet down and not to raise your knees above a comfortable height. To increase the intensity, swing your arms as you march along, and be sure your abdominals are pulled in, your head is high, and your chest is open. Do this exercise for a couple of minutes until you feel slightly warmer.

Cool-down Exercises

The cool-down is particularly important in aerobics. Chances are you've gotten your body temperature raised more doing the cardiovascular workout. You can begin your cool-down by marching in place, and then beginning to slow it down.

■ Pelvic Rock/Pelvic Tilt

Assume an all-fours position, on your hands and knees. Think of holding your back in its natural alignment (see **FIGURE 5-7**, p. 61). Then tuck only your pelvis in, bringing your pubic bone toward your neck. Be sure to move only your pelvis (see **FIGURE 5-8**, p. 61). If it helps, have someone hold your pelvis so that you can learn to isolate this area. You need to do two sets of twenty repetitions of the pelvic tilts.

■ Side Lying Stretches

Lying on your right side, stretch your right arm over your body as if reaching for something above your head. Focus on extending the arm as well as the leg and body (see **FIGURE 5-14**, p. 65). This should feel like a good tension release. Hold this pose for about ten seconds. Repeat on the left side.

■ Full Body Extension

Lying on your back, extend your arms above your head and lengthen your legs, much like the side lying extension. Hold this pose for ten seconds and repeat. You can then choose a position for relaxation.

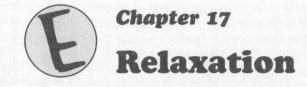

Chapter 17

Relaxation

As you learn to exercise your body, so you must learn to exercise your mind. Relaxation can be done by anyone, in any location. The benefits are amazing for the body and soul. Pregnancy is a very beneficial time to learn the techniques of relaxation to aid you throughout life.

Stress and Pregnancy

Stress is something that we have come to expect as a society. Everywhere you go people are rushing. We learn vocabulary words like *multitasking* and *pressure headaches*. We learn that time is of the essence. Time is money. Stress is no longer a "four-letter word," but a societal ideal to which we are slaves.

During pregnancy the stresses of the physical body are many. You may spend a lot of time, effort, and even money to rid yourself of the physical problems that can be associated with pregnancy. When you add the mental and emotional stress of pregnancy to the physical stresses, the physical and non-physical tension can be intense.

There are many signs that scream to you that your body is under stress:

- Headaches
- Tightness in your body
- Clenching teeth
- Restlessness
- Insomnia
- Fatigue
- Blood pressure problems
- Heartburn and other intestinal disorders
- Weight loss or gain

Why Stress Relief Is Important

No matter how you slice it, stress does not paint a pretty picture for your body. The tolls of stress on the non-pregnant body are slightly easier to recover from. However, during pregnancy the added toll of stress to your already taxed system has the potential to cause problems with the pregnancy in extreme situations.

Increased levels of stress can also affect how you absorb your nutrients, and prevent or restrict blood flow through the placenta to your baby, causing fetal growth restriction. Stress can affect how you bond prenatally with your baby. Untreated stress can make life changes more difficult, particularly those you are trying to change for the benefit of your baby, for example, quitting smoking or changing eating habits.

Even if your stress levels have not reached the extremes required to harm the pregnancy, the stress you experience can make pregnancy more difficult for you. This has led to a huge increase in stress relief products and programs.

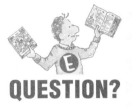

QUESTION?

What's the big deal about stress in labor?
Stress in labor has some very negative effects on the progress of labor. Nature and science tell us that if you are stressed in labor your body produces more stress hormones, cathecholamines. This can lead to a slow down of labor or a stop, called *dystocia*.

Stress relief happens in a variety of ways. From the physical to the mental, it is important to our well-being. One of the easiest ways to reduce stress is through relaxation. There are several types of relaxation and each one plays a part in your total body makeup. To neglect a component of this organization is to neglect your body. The three forms of relaxation are mental, emotional, and physical.

Mental Relaxation

Mental relaxation is probably the most widely talked about form of relaxation. If you are taking childbirth classes, you may have gone into great detail on this form of relaxation. Basically, the definition of mental relaxation is to be able to clear your mind of intrusive thoughts during certain periods.

The benefits of being able mentally to let go of ideas and extraneous thoughts is fairly obvious. You can clear your mind to deal with whatever it is you are currently doing. This type of relaxation is a *focal point*, to borrow a term from Lamaze, for many programs, including childbirth classes.

There are many ways to deal with mental stress. The one that is most available to you will probably be education. While education may sound like a simple answer to a complex problem, it is very often all you will need to help address the issues you are facing mentally in pregnancy.

If you are a fact- or detail-oriented person, this may not be a difficult task for you. Perhaps you've signed up for every class your birthing place offers. Maybe you've read some books on the topic. Chances are you've sought out some form of information about pregnancy, labor, and parenting to help you cope with the mental stresses of the unknowns. Even if this is not your first pregnancy, the issues of adding an additional person to your family or the stresses of things you would like to change from your first pregnancy can be many.

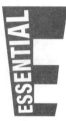

Mental relaxation can be one of the most difficult things to train your body to accomplish. Many women, particularly during pregnancy, feel like their minds are racing a hundred miles a minute. If you experience this feeling, it can lead you to a feeling of the inability to turn your brain off long enough to feel relaxed.

Emotional Relaxation

Emotional relaxation is the second hardest form of relaxation to learn. As the term implies, it has to do with dealing with the emotional issues that are affecting your life. During pregnancy, the emotional issues are many. Add hormones to the mix and you've got an interesting pot of feelings to deal with.

You might be dealing with issues of becoming a parent for the first time. This leaves you revisiting issues of your childhood, both positive and negative. You may start to look at other parents you know and wonder what type of parents you and your partner will be.

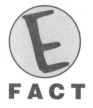

The fear-tension-pain cycle is another childbirth education backbone. This theory states that if you have fear, you tense. If you tense, you will have more pain. If you have more pain, you will fear labor and pain. The goal of most forms of relaxation taught in these classes is to interrupt the cycle and, therefore, provide pain relief.

Physical Relaxation

Contrary to popular belief, physical relaxation is much easier to achieve than mental or emotional relaxation. Your body's reaction to physical issues can be dealt with in a much clearer and more precise manner. The tools you have available to you are numerous and should be used as often as you wish. Some examples of these tools include:

- Massage
- Aromatherapy
- Music
- Acupuncture
- Hydrotherapy

Many of these tools can be used in conjunction with one another. For example, during a massage you may use some scented oils to aid in your relaxation or perhaps you listen to the radio while you take a bath or shower. Sometimes you use these tools without being aware of their use or that you are deriving benefits from them. Think of how you feel when one of your favorite songs comes on the radio. First, you might tap your toes or fingers, but before you know it you are singing along, even when it is not necessarily appropriate. This is your body responding positively to something you enjoy. Your body responds with the production of endorphins, hormones that make you naturally feel pleasant and relaxed.

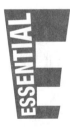

No matter what types of concerns you have or how confident you are in previous parenting skills, you have a lot to deal with during this pregnancy. The stress that comes from these issues cannot be answered simply. The good news is that the relaxation exercises can help you deal with these problems both in the physical and mental forms.

While these tools are available for your use, even during pregnancy, they are not necessary for physical relaxation. They should be looked at merely as aids in the relaxation process. You will learn some physical relaxation techniques later in the chapter, such as the tense-release exercises, that use only your own body versus choosing to incorporate your partner into your physical relaxation for assistance. Do whatever makes you feel comfortable. Exercise is one of the best ways to deal with the physical stresses of life.

Exercise and Stress Relief

Exercise has always been a great way to deal with stress. Not only are there the obvious physical benefits of exercise, but now we are starting to recognize the stress-relieving benefits as well. In fact, many health-care providers recommend exercise as the number-one method of stress relief.

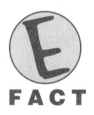

FACT

Using exercise to help your body rid itself of physical tension is an easy way to deal with stress on a simple level. Even on days you don't feel well, simple exercises can help you feel better by elevating your body's natural levels of endorphins and other pleasant-feeling hormones.

Distraction Techniques

Distraction techniques do just what they promise—they distract you. The best pregnancy based example I can offer is patterned paced breathing for labor. By focusing on your breathing rather than contractions, you use your mind to focus on something other than the contractions and discomfort. When practiced diligently it works really well, but practice is the key. This type of relaxation is beneficial for you if you harbor fear or tension related to a process or if escape is a common coping technique for you in life, in general.

The breath focusing of patterned paced breathing is used in many forms. One technique is to focus on the in and out breaths as you breathe. You can do this easily by slowly counting to ten and breathing in through your mouth. Hold that breath for a few comfortable seconds and then release your breath to the count of ten through your nose. If you find that ten seconds is too long, or too short, feel free to alter this number to whatever works well for you. Some also find that they prefer mouth breathing or nose breathing, so use whatever method of breathing feels natural to you.

This is but one example of a distraction technique. There are many others that you can use to help aid in relaxation throughout life. Some require even less thought than breathing, like listening to music, or watching movies or television. Many times you become so familiar with whatever method you choose that when a stressful situation comes up you do not even realize that you have reverted to doing your distraction technique.

Internal Focus Techniques

Through internal focus, you can directly address concerns about your body by using your mind. The benefit of using an internal focus can be that you are able to focus directly on your situation. Many of these techniques are used in childbirth classes and include focusing on the thoughts associated with the processes you are going through. These techniques work really well for you if you are fact-focused and interested in learning everything you can. This can also help alleviate fears associated with certain processes.

ALERT!

Although it sounds like something you would know not to do, be very careful about using relaxation tapes of even soothing music while driving your car. Much like the warnings found on narcotics, keep in mind that these exercises can have a powerful effect on your reflexes and alertness.

Mental Imagery

Mental imagery is simply defined as the ability to "see" images or scenes. This practice is used as a coping mechanism that can either be distracting or an internal focus. These techniques are used by many athletes before competition to improve performance.

Labor, birth, and parenting are no less of a performance and using these techniques can greatly enhance your coping mechanisms. The techniques can also be used in conjunction with nearly any type of birth experience and do not depend on your physical status.

Common types of mental images used in birth are those that are open and flowing. You can use waves to imagine a contraction pattern. You might use the image of a flower opening, like a rose bud, to imagine what your cervix is doing during labor.

The Perfect Memory

Many people choose to use a time and place that they have actually experienced to aid them in their relaxation. Using this mental imagery is very beneficial. You can choose any time or place that provides you with a positive memory. Be sure to recall as many physical and emotional details as possible. Things to remember include what you were wearing, who you were with, who said what, what smells were around you, what time of day or year it was. Was it a special occasion?

You can choose a variety of situations, like your most romantic memory, a great vacation, a family getaway, and so forth. Is your memory perhaps merely a favorite place? A childhood safe haven or vacation home often works well. The key is to choose something or someplace that makes you feel good and safe.

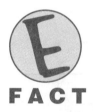

FACT

By using the mental images of winning a competition or even competing, it can actually reduce the tension and stress felt when the competition arrives. People who do public speaking also use similar techniques to help reduce anxiety about their performances.

The Birth Exercise

Using mental imagery to conjure up the birth of your baby can be a valuable tool. Simply use techniques to picture what you would like to happen during this special time. You might incorporate some of the facts you've learned about your body and childbirth in general to help you imagine your baby's birth. This also gives you the ideal time and place to work through your fears and concerns.

To do this exercise, get in a relaxing position and set the mood with music and lighting if desired. Start with how you imagine your labor beginning and slowly proceed through the birth as you see it happening. If there is something or someplace where you get "stuck" and can't envision, do not panic, move on. It will come. You can end at any point. Some end their imaginings with the birth of the baby, so you might choose to end there or a bit further postpartum.

This mental rehearsing is a great way to prepare yourself for the experience, even though it is not likely to go exactly as you have imagined it. It will also help reduce your prenatal anxiety and the stresses you feel once labor has begun. You can also do this with your husband or partner. Allow him or her to tell you the story of the birth while you focus on the physical relaxation. This can help you work through differences the two of you have in philosophy or experience. Don't hesitate to say how you imagine it all working out.

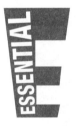

Touring the hospital or birth center you intend to give birth at can greatly reduce your levels of fear and anxiety associated with birth. It not only allows you to actually see the facility and learn about their procedures and protocols, but it can also enable you to rehearse mentally how everything will happen once it's your turn to give birth.

Tense-Release Exercises

Tense-release exercises are the most basic form of physical relaxation. You probably use these techniques without even realizing that you are doing them. Clenching your fists and relaxing them, for example, is something many of us do if we're angry. Perhaps when you feel a tension headache coming on, you might scrunch your neck up and then extend it a bit. These are all tense-release exercises.

You can use the tense-release technique consciously to help alleviate tension in muscles throughout your pregnancy. One of the great things about tense-release exercises is that they can be done in nearly any situation. These can even be done if you experience complications.

To do a formal tense-release exercise, assume a comfortable position;

this can be sitting or lying down. You can set the mood with music or dimmed lighting if you desire. Start at the top of your body—your head. Scrunch your forehead up as tightly as you can. Hold the tension for up to five seconds. Then, deliberately release the tension from your forehead. Experience the difference between the tension previously felt and the current state of relaxation. Invite your partner or coach to experience your tension and relaxation both visually and by the use of touch. This will help him or her guide you in labor.

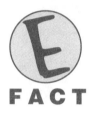

FACT

Stretching is a form of tense-release exercise. Typically, the goal of stretching prior to exercise is to release tension and warm up muscles prior to exercise. This would be a good example of using tension versus relaxation as a benefit to your workout and your stress levels.

Next, go lower and scrunch your face and ears. Hold for five seconds and release. Now tighten your neck so that your ears rest on your shoulders. Hold this for an additional five seconds and again release. Tighten your back, holding for five seconds and releasing. Now do the same with your arms and hands, holding the tension for five seconds and releasing the tension. Next scrunch your buttocks and hips; hold for five and release. Proceed to do the same with your thighs, and then your lower legs and feet.

For an added "workout," have your partner massage you to help you learn to release the tension. To do this, simply have your partner begin to massage the tensed area three to four seconds into the holding phase of the tension. You can also make a game of this by trying to hide tension and making your partner find it.

Touch Therapy and Massage

Touch is usually a very positive thing for most people, so when you add to that the benefits of touch on healing and physical and emotional well-being, we know that the benefits are many. Massage is commonly used in athletics as a form of physical therapy, but it can also be used to relax and ease the mental and physical stressors of pregnancy.

The physical benefits of massage on pregnancy are numerous. Massage can help alleviate or prevent muscle aches and strains associated with physical changes in your body or exercise-related issues. It can also help increase and improve your circulation, a must when your pregnant body is dealing with an ever-expanding blood volume. It can also help with swelling issues and problems related to stress, such as insomnia and blood pressure concerns.

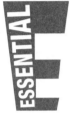

If you think massage is great for you, try it for your baby! Take a class in infant massage with your newborn and learn about benefits like less gas and colic, more peaceful rest, and just a great time with your new little one as you learn to respond to their needs and cues.

Massage can be done at nearly any point in pregnancy. Some massage practitioners will schedule massages in blocks of time from fifteen to seventy-five minutes depending on your personal needs. You can also set your own schedule for how often you receive massage. There is no one right answer for how often you can or should have a massage.

Finding a Massage Practitioner

There are many organizations that certify or train massage therapy practitioners. Some actually offer certifications in pregnancy and the childbearing year. You should always interview the person you are working with, even if it is someone you have been seeing for years, about their knowledge of pregnancy and its related issues.

Your massage therapist should be forthcoming about his or her training. Some may even request a specific release from your doctor or midwife to allow you to continue receiving massages throughout pregnancy. Some practitioners of massage will not perform massages on women who are less than twelve weeks' gestation. While massage has never been implicated in early miscarriage, it is important to talk to your doctor or midwife and your massage therapist about concerns related to your physical well-being in pregnancy.

ALERT!

It is important that you find a practitioner who is trained to deal with pregnant women. There are certain points in your body and certain types of massage that you do not want in pregnancy. If someone is not trained, they can actually harm you during pregnancy. An example would be certain acupressure points near your ankles that can stimulate early contractions.

Your Massage Experience

If you have never had a massage before, you might be wondering what actually happens during a massage. Part of what happens will depend on the type and length of massage, as well as your practitioner and your comfort levels. Generally speaking, massage is performed with you lying down on a special table, with a section cut out for your expanding abdomen, or with your body propped on pillow bolsters to prevent you from lying on your back. The room usually has dimmed lighting to promote relaxation. There may also be candles or aromatherapy to add to the effects.

ESSENTIAL

As pregnant women are very sensitive to smells, never hesitate to tell your therapist how the smells she is using affect you. You can even bring your own scents or request unscented lotions should the smells be aggravating to your senses.

Many therapists have you remove your clothing completely or down to the underwear, no bra. That said, there is a sheet and/or blanket used to cover you the entire massage. Some forms of massage are done over the blanket to ensure your privacy, while still providing you with the best massage physically. Removing clothing is obviously not acceptable for all, and again is something you need to discuss with the practitioner.

Partner Massage

Professional massage, while nice, is not for everyone. You may, therefore, choose to supplement visits with your massage therapist with massages from your partner, or even a good friend. These are great stress relievers, particularly at the end of the day.

Suggest to your partner that you practice some of the relaxation techniques you have learned prior to bed each night. This has the added benefits of relaxing you mentally and physically and can help you sleep more soundly.

Do not be fearful of how to massage someone. The techniques are easy to learn. Many childbirth classes incorporate massage into their class schedules because the benefit is so great. If you haven't yet signed up for a class, just tell your partner what feels good or what is hurting. Massage tends to be a pretty instinctual experience. If the massage you receive isn't exactly what you need, offer to massage your partner the way you'd like to be massaged. This usually gets the message across very efficiently.

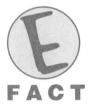

FACT

While a massage sounds great, you may be thinking you simply don't have the time. Try a quick massage of either your hands or feet done with a partner or by yourself to help relieve tension and prevent common problems of pregnancy like carpal tunnel syndrome.

As you see, relaxation is a key to understanding the body's processes throughout life and particularly during pregnancy. As stress can have a negative impact on your physical, mental, and emotional well-being, you need to be aware of the tension that can gather in your body. Using the tools discussed in this chapter, you can reduce the negative effects of stress and tension on your mind and body. This will also help prepare you for the roller coaster of parenting. (E)

Chapter 18

Exercise in Special Situations

Even if you have done everything perfectly, you might be one of the few women who experiences a pregnancy complication. Some of these complications can alter your plans for a physical pregnancy. If this happens, there are solutions to help you maintain muscles, relieve stress, and deal effectively with the complications you are facing.

When You Can't Exercise Regularly

The majority of pregnancies will proceed without any complications. If you find that your pregnancy is one of the few that requires restrictions on your physical expenditures, then you will need help in dealing with the added complications of the lack of physical movement.

Sometimes your practitioner will ask you to reduce or remove exercise from your daily pregnancy schedule. You may be asked to keep this restriction for only a few weeks, until a specific problem clears up, or for the remainder of the pregnancy. This is the least restrictive form of pregnancy modification.

Bed Rest

Bed rest can be prescribed for your pregnancy to help prevent problems or complications. It can be prescribed early in pregnancy or late in pregnancy, and can last anywhere from a few days to months. Some conditions that may require some form of bed rest might be:

- Placenta previa
- Preterm labor
- Cerclage or premature dilation
- Multiple gestation (particularly higher order multiples)
- Fetal growth restriction

Moderate Bed Rest

Moderate bed rest is often prescribed for mild complications of pregnancy such as elevated blood pressure or a threatened early miscarriage. Typically, this form of bed rest doesn't last very long. If you are placed on moderate bed rest, you will probably be given very clear indications of how much you should be up and around. You may have a certain number of hours that you are required to stay in bed.

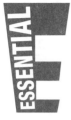

Support is crucial in a pregnancy that requires bed rest. Whether you have children at home or you don't, look into having friends and family help with housework, chores, and meals while you're resting to protect your baby. Many are glad to lend a hand. If that's not possible, find professional support through the use of a postpartum doula (✍ *www.dona.org*).

Strict Bed Rest

Strict bed rest is the second highest form of bed rest. This is prescribed for complications, such as active bleeding from placenta previa and preterm labor, which is controlled through rest or medications. If you are on strict bed rest, you might be asked to stay in bed except for a certain list of things you do daily. This can include bathroom breaks, a shower or bath, and perhaps one meal with your family.

Hospital Bed Rest

Hospital bed rest is the most severe form of bed rest. It is used for complications with preterm labor that are not well controlled. It can also be used if you are prematurely dilating or if your bag of waters (membranes) has ruptured, prior to term. You may even be forced to use a bed pan or catheter to use the bathroom. Sometimes you will be kept in bed at an angle, called *Trendelenberg position*, where your head is kept below your feet. While this is uncomfortable, it is used to remove pressure from your cervix. Generally, you will stay here until the birth of your baby.

Physical Activity and Bed Rest

Bed rest can be a vital part of your pregnancy care. Even if you are on the strictest form of bed rest, exercise can be vital. There are some simple exercises that can help you. The lack of physical activity, on the other hand, can have a detrimental effect on your body physically, mentally, and emotionally. This must be weighed against the hazards of activity on your pregnancy, your baby, and your body.

The biggest fear of bed rest is that your body will physically atrophy to the point where you are unable to resume a normal activity level after the birth. When physical inactivity is necessary, this can cause your muscles to lose their tone. The lack of routine weight bearing can also cause calcium loss from your bones. The effect on your body is a feeling of weakness and inability to get around.

E ALERT!

Left-sided bed rest is thought to be the best position to bring nutrients and oxygen to your baby. The blood flow to the placenta is supposedly enhanced by this position. This allows your baby a better chance at obtaining what he or she needs to grow. The only really bad position would be the supine or back lying position.

If you are on a less severe form of bed rest, start making plans for physical activity by talking to your practitioner about simple stretches. These do not raise your heart rate but do offer your muscle some form of exercise and tension relief. Simple stretches can be done even while in bed if necessary.

Communicating with Your Practitioner

During this emotionally difficult time in your pregnancy, your doctor or midwife will be your main source of support and information. This relationship is key to you and your baby's health. This is why the trust you have spent the earlier part of your pregnancy developing is so important.

If you were physically active before pregnancy, the thought of being inactive may truly scare you. Even when faced with potential negative complications with your pregnancy or to your health, you may still be concerned about this lack of exercise. By talking to your practitioner, you can learn why restrictions are necessary and what you can do about them. Sometimes the restrictions are temporary, but other times they are not. Dealing with this will be something you will need a lot of support in resolving. Your practitioner will help you answer these questions.

Your practitioner may have certain tricks in his or her bag to help alleviate your fears. It is to his or her advantage that you are emotionally adjusted to the new reality of your pregnancy. He also has a vested interest in keeping you, and subsequently, your baby, healthy. Sometimes this involves minor stretching exercises that you can do, perhaps even isometrics and other forms of exercise. The nurses and other educators can also help you find resources. Another place to look for help would be the physical therapy department.

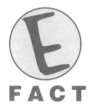

FACT

Sidelines (✍ *www.sidelines.org*) is a national organization to support families on bed rest. If you are on bed rest, consider looking to Sidelines for support. They have a variety of programs including peer counseling, a Web site with forums and bed rest chats, and publications with helpful tips for making the most of bed rest or restricted activity.

Physical Therapy

The physical therapy department may be what you think of when you see people who have been in debilitating car wrecks or accidents of some form. However, these specially trained therapists are specialists in the human body and its functions. Your doctor or midwife can help you find a therapist to assist you with body work either in the hospital or at home on bed rest.

The physical therapy would usually consist of simple exercises done with the therapist, even when large movements or being out of bed is out of the question. The benefits of using physical therapy include counteracting many of the negative outcomes of bed rest—including muscular atrophy and calcium depletion in your bones—and simply feeling better. The more you maintain during your period of bed rest, the better you will be in the short term and postpartum.

If you think physical therapy can help you and no one has mentioned it to you, do not hesitate to ask for a referral from your practitioner. Being proactive in your health care can only make you and your baby healthier. If your practitioner doesn't know of someone or can't find someone who specializes in pregnancy, ask a local high-risk center, the local physical therapy association, or organizations such as Sidelines for a referral in your area.

Maintaining Muscle

You may firmly believe that exercise is appropriate in pregnancy. You may also believe that building muscle in pregnancy is appropriate. In general, the maintenance of muscle is what should be the goal of pregnancy fitness. When complications arise in your pregnancy, this is definitely where your focus should be shifted.

It is important to remember that muscles are simple fibers made up of protein. They simply contract and lengthen. Lack of use will make them weak, but it will not turn them into fat. The muscles you have cannot be converted to fatty tissue.

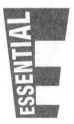

"Massage can have a definite benefit for the woman on bed rest," says Laura Davis, RN and massage therapist specializing in pregnancy, postpartum, and newborn massage. "It can help alleviate stress on the muscles and generally allow the mother to feel better about her body and her situation through physical contact."

Using the resistance exercises of a physical therapist and stretching designed for women in your situation, you can hope to maintain at least some of the muscle mass you have attained prior to pregnancy. While the loss of muscle is not a good thing, there is a common-sense trade-off between maintaining a healthy pregnancy and maintaining muscle. It is a question for you and your practitioner to answer: where you and your pregnancy lie in that continuum.

Exercise with a Multiple Pregnancy

Multiple pregnancies are on the rise in the last ten to twenty years. The good news is that if you find yourself faced with a multiple pregnancy, so much more is known about the physical and mental aspects of multiple pregnancies than in past years. The research has included how exercise can play a beneficial role in your multiple pregnancy.

Your multiple pregnancy can be more prone to normal physical pregnancy complications like a separation of the rectus muscles in the abdomen. You will also be expected to gain more weight and eat more protein for the nourishment of your additional passenger. Your balance is likely to be affected earlier. You will likely feel more pelvic floor pressure and be more likely to suffer from physical complaints like backache, shortness of breath, and other physical complaints of pregnancy. These also tend to happen earlier.

Most practitioners agree that your exercise levels will be best served by your ability to listen to your body. Fatigue and other symptoms of a normal pregnancy are exacerbated by multiples. If you are able to rest when your body says rest, and to follow your instincts, you will probably have no additional restrictions. This will usually mean that by the second trimester you have slowed down considerably. Your third trimester will usually see an even greater slowing down in activity.

Twin Pregnancy

The majority of women experiencing a multiple pregnancy are carrying twins. Twin births occur about once in every eighty-nine births. This most common form of multiple pregnancies is also the most widely studied. Higher order multiples, or super twins, are more rare but are when there are triplets, quadruplets, or more. The more babies you are pregnant with, the more likely you are to have severe restrictions on your activity levels in pregnancy. As with any complication or situation in pregnancy, your communication with your practitioner is very important.

If you are expecting twins, chances are you will have very few restrictions on your pregnancy exercise routine, compared to higher order multiples. You will, however, be more carefully monitored. The risks associated with your twin pregnancy will include the higher risk of preterm labor and birth. While exercise may have nothing to do with this risk, it is important to know the signs.

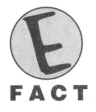

FACT

Nutrition is always an important subject in pregnancy. When you find yourself on bed rest, it becomes even more important. Talk to your practitioner about finding a dietician, someone who has special training in nutrition, to help you maintain the adequate amount of calories for your special pregnancy and its unique needs.

Stretch Exercises

Since stretching is probably what you will likely be able to do on the stricter forms of bed rest, you should look at stretching as a good form of stress relief and physical exercise. The key to getting the most out of your stretch routines will be doing them only to the point of comfort. You wish to do all of the movement on your exhale. Remember to adjust the number of repetitions downward if you find yourself getting tired.

Seated Stretches

Some of these stretches require you to be seated, whereas others can be done while lying down in bed. For an extra position, try some of these while in the bathtub. It's your own mini-version of water exercise. The benefit? You have slight added resistance from the water in the tub.

ESSENTIAL

If your doctor, midwife, or physical therapist agrees, try using very light weights draped over your ankles or wrists while doing some of the exercises. You can fill a large tube sock with a pound of rice and allow half the sock to hang on either side. Your goal is not to apply a huge amount of weight, but to have some form of resistance.

■ Shoulder Rounds

Without changing the position of your body, try to exaggerate a shrug upward with your shoulders, bringing them to your ears. Hold this position for five to ten seconds. Then relax your shoulders back to their beginning position. Move your shoulders in small circles forward for ten repetitions, and then reverse and go backward for ten repetitions.

■ Seated Leg Lifts

Sit on the edge of your bed. Allow both of your feet to hang over the side. It is not necessary that your legs touch the ground. Drape the sock weight over your right ankle. Slowly raise the right leg as you exhale (see **FIGURE 11-1**, p. 159). Do not bring your leg up to the point of pain, and it should not be raised higher than knee level. Slowly lower your leg. Repeat this for a count of ten repetitions on each leg.

Standing Stretches

If you are on a stricter form of bed rest, these exercises may not be appropriate for you. Standing can increase the pressure on your cervix. If the reason you are on bed rest is to decrease that pressure, you will most likely not be able to use the standing or even some of the seated exercises.

■ Middle Chest Stretch

With your feet about shoulder-width apart, place your hands on your lower back, just above your buttocks. Slowly begin to stretch backward as you try to pull your shoulder blades and elbows together. Hold this pose for about five to ten seconds. Repeat the stretch up to ten times. Be sure to keep your chin level and your head facing forward. Always tuck in your abdominal muscles.

■ Calf Stretch

With your hands on your hips and your feet shoulder-width apart, point your toes forward (see **FIGURE 7-3**, p. 100). Step backward with your right foot. The step length should be comfortable and yet a stretch. Ensuring your posture is aligned properly, lean forward, making sure your knee does not extend over your foot (see **FIGURE 7-4**, p. 100). This stretch will be felt in the calf of your rear leg. Do ten of these repetitions and then repeat on the opposite side.

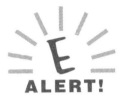

ALERT!

If you find yourself in need of some stability while you do any of these exercises, always use some form of support—use a chair placed to one side to hang on to, or even the wall in front of you. It is important to remember about the balance issue during pregnancy.

■ Chest Stretch

Stand with your feet about shoulder-width apart, pelvis tucked in and abdominals held tightly. Spread your arms to each side, at shoulder level (see **FIGURE 6-3**, p. 79). Slowly curl your back forward, while bringing your arms forward as well. Allow your head to go forward slowly with this motion but try to keep the tension from your neck (see **FIGURE 6-4**, p. 79). As you return to a standing pose, spread your arms back to your side and feel the stretch in your chest. To ensure you feel this stretch, pull your shoulder blades together behind your back. Repeat this for ten repetitions.

■ Upward Stretch

Stand with your feet about hip-distance apart, with your left hand on the left hip. Reach your opposite arm slowly up over your head. To prevent balance problems, try to keep your arm slightly forward of your body. If you still have trouble with balance, step forward slightly with your right foot. Do up to ten repetitions on each side.

■ Side Stretch

With your feet hip-width apart, let your arms hang by your sides. Hold your head up and imagine your spine lengthening. Slowly bend from your waist to the right side of your body. You can hold your right arm slightly away from your body or you can slide that arm down your leg (see **FIGURE 6-5**, p. 80). Your left arm can be held away from your body to help you balance if you need it. This will help prevent you from leaning back, which can cause backache as your abdomen grows. Slowly return to a standing position. Do one on each side (alternating) for a total of twenty repetitions.

■ Upper Back Stretch

Sit on the birth ball with your feet facing forward in front of you. Lift your arms above your head, palms facing forward. Extend your upper back, one vertebra at a time (see **FIGURE 6-6**, p. 81). As you feel your spine lengthen, you will be stretching your upper back. Now relax one arm to the side, and do each arm singly. Repeat ten times on each side and finish with both arms stretching again.

Stress Relief Exercises

You are lying in bed on bed rest. You can't get up, even to go to the bathroom. While this may not be the ideal situation, you realize it is what your baby needs to continue to grow inside your body. The good news is that there are still things you can do to help exercise, even when movement is the last thing you are supposed to do.

ESSENTIAL

Using the tense-relax techniques will teach you to be able to recognize tension in your body. This additional knowledge will help you throughout your life. Unfortunately, tension and stress is a part of life we must learn to deal with. Dealing with it is preferable to learning to live with it.

Breath Focusing

One technique is to focus on the in and out breaths as you breathe. You can do this easily by slowly counting to ten and breathing in through your mouth. Hold that breath for a few, comfortable seconds and then release your breath to the count of ten through your nose. If you find that ten seconds is too long or short, feel free to alter this number to whatever works well for you. Some also find that they prefer mouth breathing to nose breathing, so use whatever method of breathing feels natural to you.

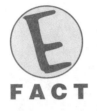

FACT

Learning to take it easy while exercising is an important part of exercising. Just as you have days when you feel good and days when you don't feel good, you will have off days during pregnancy. These days are days to kick back and relax. Your baby and your body will thank you.

Mental Imagery

The relaxation exercises you have learned will also help aid you in preventing added tension to your body. Focusing on nurturing mental imagery and a healthy outcome for you and your baby are imperative.

Mental imagery can be done in nearly any form, at any location, even on strict bed rest. If, for example, you are having problems with your cervix dilating prematurely, visualize the cervix closing and holding your baby in until an appropriate time to be born. Perhaps the impending birth is only a matter of days away and your concern is the lung maturity of your baby. Imagine the medications you've had strengthening your baby's lungs. "Watch" your baby practice breathing movements.

Chapter 19

Postpartum: The First Few Days

Congratulations! Your baby is here! Adjusting to life after birth is a big deal. You have many physical changes, including the sudden drop in hormones. You also have a new little one or ones to deal with. All of these changes can alter how you view your life and your body.

Your New Body

The first few minutes after birth may leave you in awe of everything that is going on. Your body has just amazingly given birth to this little creature. Now your breasts are primed and ready to make milk to continue its nurturing process. This is a special bonding time for the whole family.

After you have taken a while to notice the many changes about you, your focus may turn inward. The nurses or assistants help you learn how to take care of your postpartum body as it goes through many changes. You start to explore your new body. You might even be relieved at how light you feel.

The Physical Changes

One of the first physical differences you may notice is your breathing. After having spent many months in tight quarters, your lungs and diaphragm can now expand. You may have spent much of the last few months dreaming about the ability to breathe deeply again. While it may physically be possible now, it is not as comfortable as you might think. Many women report that breathing deeply can cause a sore feeling as the organs shift back. Thankfully, this feeling usually lasts no more than a few hours. Deep breathing is recommended to help alleviate this pain.

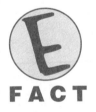

FACT

Stretch marks earned during pregnancy have not gone away, but they will be much less noticeable. The further you get from your pregnancy, the less noticeable they are. The first thing to go will be the bright red, angry color. Over time these badges of motherhood will fade to barely visible silver lines.

You might also be anxious to explore your now-deflated abdomen. The good news is that the baby is now residing on the outside. The surprising news is that your abdomen is not flat. The skin has been stretched, over the period of months. It will take time to get it back to any shape or previous tone. Some exercises can help speed this process, but not by much time.

When you first get out of bed, you may find that you are shaky on your feet. Be sure to get up with some help and take your time. You should not try to carry your baby. This can be due to many factors. If you haven't eaten for a long period of time, your shakiness may be helped by a meal. If you are experiencing the shakes, which are very normal and occur no matter how you gave birth, try warm blankets to ease this discomfort.

Your breasts are not much different. That is because they have been preparing for this day for many months. Your breasts have been ready to produce breast milk since about the sixteenth week of pregnancy. The birth of your baby does signal your breasts to start the transition from colostrum, your first milk, to mature milk. It will take three to seven days for your milk to come in.

The First Exercises after Birth

Believe it or not, the best time to begin exercise is immediately after birth. As soon as you remember, begin to think about doing exercises. You have just completed a marathon, and while you do need rest, there are certain exercises that can help you heal.

You might wonder why this is so important. Exercise has numerous benefits to the postpartum mother, including:

- Sense of well-being
- Weight loss
- Reduction in stress
- Fewer sleep problems associated with stress
- Return to a semblance of normal
- Reduction in baby blues and possibly postpartum depression
- Fewer feelings of isolation, particularly if doing group exercises

Kegels

The pelvic floor exercises that were so important before giving birth are even more important now. Remember, these perineal exercises will help increase the blood flow to that area, which will help speed the healing process and relieve pain.

At first you may have trouble isolating the muscles. This is common and you should not worry. Even if you required no stitches or sutures, the area still has been stretched to allow your baby to be born. If you did require stitches, whether or not an episiotomy was performed, you can still safely do these exercises.

ALERT!

The American Academy of Pediatrics recommends that you begin breastfeeding within the first thirty minutes of birth when possible. It is thought that this first nursing, prior to your baby's first deep sleep, imprints the correct nursing ability on their minds—not to mention that the first milk, colostrum, contains some wonderful antibodies to help protect your baby from illness and intestinal problems.

Begin by doing simple flicks. You do not need to hold the counts. Merely tightening and releasing will be helpful to your recovery. You can gradually increase what you do as you feel comfortable. It is generally not recommend that you sit on a doughnut or other inflated cushion. You should continue to sit on hard surfaces. Sit evenly, not leaning to one side or the other. You should also avoid crossing your legs, even at the ankle. This can cause your perineum to heal inappropriately, particularly if you had stitches.

Pain in this area will begin to subside and gradually get better each day. If you had stitches, they generally dissolve and do not require any special care. By the end of six weeks, your bottom should be feeling as good as new. If it isn't, be sure to talk to your doctor or midwife at your six-week checkup.

Abdominal Tightening

Abdominal tightening is a very simple exercise. It offers you the benefit of beginning to heal the abdominal muscles. It also provides you with more awareness of this area. The sooner you begin working on this, the sooner your abdomen heals and returns close to its original state.

Abdominal tightening is done simply by thinking about sucking in your abdomen. Think of pulling your belly button all the way back to your spine. Do this as you inhale. Hold the "stretch" for a few seconds, and then slowly exhale. You can do five to ten repetitions of this exercise whenever you think about it. This encourages stretched muscle fibers to shorten.

Breathing

It sounds simple, right? Breathe . . . we've been telling you to do that for a long time. This time breathing has a different focus—healing. Each deep breath you take not only helps reinflate your lungs and oxygenate your body, but it enables you to heal and recover by preventing some complications of postpartum.

ESSENTIAL

Breathing after a cesarean can be painful. Even a small amount of phlegm can cause you to prefer choking to death rather than breathing. If you had a cesarean, you might even be given a breathing machine that is like a video game. You will have to blow hard enough to make a ball rise to the top of a canister.

Postpartum Pain Relief Remedies

Pain is expected after you give birth. Your body was involved in a major physical activity and needs to react to the changes. There are many things you can do for pain relief. Cold packs should be used during the first twelve hours. This helps reduce the swelling. Some maxi pads come with cold packs built in. If you do not have access to these, ask the nurse to help you make a cold pack using gloves or a baggy and some ice. Be careful not to apply ice directly to the area. The goal is not to cause freezer burn, but to help reduce the swelling in the tissues.

You can also try a sitz bath. This is done by allowing warm water to pass over your perineum. Some hospitals or birth centers have special tubs or chairs designed for this. There is also a portable sitz bath available that you can use at home. If you have access to either, fill your home bathtub with about 6 inches of warm water. You can soak, but not bathe, in this water.

There are also commercial preparations or salves that you can add to your sitz bath. These are usually made from herbs that promote healing to the tissues and help with pain. Talk to your practitioner about using them or get a recommendation from someone who has used one.

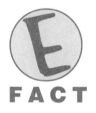

FACT

Comfrey root is a soothing herb to use on your bottom after birth. To use it, simply purchase the root and boil it in a quart of water for ten minutes. Allow the mixture to steep and then remove the herb and throw it away. The water can be used in your peri-bottle, your sitz bath, or as a compress.

There are also many medications that can be used on your bottom after birth. Witch hazel pads are commonly given out to help with pain and swelling. They can also be used for hemorrhoids. There are also a variety of creams and sprays available to use. Many contain numbing agents to anesthetize the area.

Cesarean Recovery

Even if you had a normal, uneventful pregnancy, your chance of having a cesarean is nearly one in four. Since 25 percent of women will have a cesarean in the United States, you need to be aware of your risks.

The exercises for a vaginal birth are also applicable to cesarean recovery. The focus on your breathing will be stressed, because after surgery there are some complications that you are more likely to experience, like blood clots and breathing difficulties. Breathing deeply can help prevent these.

It is also imperative that you begin walking as soon as you are able to. Your intestines will be sluggish after surgery, and walking will help increase the movement of your intestines, peristalsis, as well as decrease the time of your recovery. It also helps avoid some complications of postpartum.

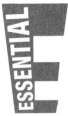

Getting up for the first time after a cesarean surgery is not fun. Find a pillow or other soft object to clutch to your abdomen. You may feel like you are going to burst or that your organs will fall out. This is normal and will pass quickly, particularly the more you get up and get moving.

After a cesarean, you will also want to limit how much weight you lift or carry. A good rule is to carry nothing heavier than your baby for a few weeks. You will also want to minimize the amount of stair climbing you do. Set up a makeshift nursery downstairs. This prevents you from being isolated in your room and yet also keeps you from taking forty treks upstairs for diapers.

Resuming Exercise

Resuming exercise has many benefits. And yet our society sends us mixed signals about what we should do and how we should act as new mothers. You might feel torn between resting and recuperating with baby and hurrying up and getting back to your "old self." Don't let these societal mixed messages push you.

It is important that you begin to pace yourself. Work on your fitness level and body awareness at your own speed. There are many factors that will go into your readiness to exercise.

The standard answer often quoted in many pregnancy books is six weeks. This rarely takes into account how you gave birth or other factors. It is important that the answer you are given be appropriate for your body, whether that be more or less time.

How you gave birth will have a significant impact on when you can resume exercising regularly. While there are always simple toning exercises that can be done, many women want to know when they can get back to their normal routines. Part of the answer will depend on if you had a normal vaginal birth, and instrumental delivery (forceps or vacuum), or whether you had a surgical birth (cesarean section).

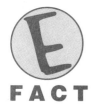

FACT

Involution is the process of your uterus shrinking and the placental site healing. A breastfeeding mother will have a faster time to involution because of the added hormones produced by her body as her baby nurses. Not only will this help you exercise sooner, but also it reduces your risks of certain postpartum complications.

Vaginal Birth

If you had a spontaneous vaginal birth, with or without any stitches, chances are you will be able to know when your body is ready to exercise again. For many women, this will be in fewer than the standard six weeks. There are a couple of things you will need to look for and do prior to beginning, even if you feel ready.

The first is to see how your bleeding is doing. Typically after any birth you will bleed, called *lochia*, for up to eight weeks after the birth. This bleeding comes from your placental site and is a measure of how healed the uterus is at any given point. This bleeding will change in color and quantity as you get further away from the birth. If your bleeding has stopped, you may be ready to exercise.

ALERT!

If you wipe and find small bits of black material on your toilet paper, do not be concerned. As the stitches reabsorb, the outside portion is sloughed off. You may notice this in your underwear, on your pad, or on the toilet paper.

Your symptoms that appeared after the birth like sweating and shaking need to have stopped. You need to feel well nourished and well hydrated before beginning any exercise program. These can be one of the most important signs.

If you feel that all of this is in order, call your practitioner. Even if you have an appointment at the six-week postpartum mark, feel free to call earlier. Explain to the doctor or midwife that you feel your body has healed well. Tell them the status of your bleeding and your general feeling. Talk to them about starting slowly and ask what signs or symptoms you should look for, so that you would know when to cease your new routine.

Instrumental Delivery

If you had an instrumental delivery, with forceps or a vacuum, you may have more healing time required. These instruments can damage internal tissues and may have required you to need more stitches than an episiotomy or tear may have required. If you meet the criteria listed, feel free to talk to your doctor or midwife. She may ask you to have your perineal area examined prior to resuming exercise. With her blessing, you may resume exercising.

Cesarean Birth

A surgical or cesarean birth is a birth, but you must also remember that it is major abdominal surgery. This surgery does cut into the abdominal muscles. This alone will increase your healing time.

You will still bleed, just as you would with a vaginal birth. This is because the bleeding does not come from the incision but rather the placental site healing. Do not be frightened about vaginal bleeding. This does frighten some women, who assume it is from the actual vaginal birth.

Your iron stores and energy in general are likely to be low after surgery. A proper diet and good nutritional intake are key to healing. You may be prescribed a certain diet or vitamins to help speed this area of healing. Eating dark leafy greens, red meats, and proteins can help you fight off low iron or anemia. This can also help you feel like you have more strength.

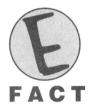

FACT

The International Cesarean Awareness Network (☞ *www.ican-online.org*) is a network designed to help women recovering from cesarean section. It can provide you with physical, mental, and emotional support after a surgical birth. There are many local chapters and peer counselors that can also help answer questions about getting your body back after abdominal surgery.

Your practitioner will be able to help you determine when you should exercise. Since you have had surgery, this may be later than other women you know who did not. Or you may simply have to go more slowly, which is never a bad idea anyway.

Fitness Level

If you were someone who was extremely fit prior to getting pregnant and you maintained a great level of fitness prior to birth, you may be ready to exercise before your other postpartum counterparts. This is also true if you had a cesarean section. A body that was well nourished and fit will recover faster, even from major surgery.

Life Factors

When it comes down to it, one of the most important factors in your readiness to begin a new fitness program after you give birth is your life. Aside from the physical factors of recovery, which will come without much help from you, you need to work on finding the time in your new schedule for exercise. Remember, consistency is the key to good exercise. It is almost more harmful not to exercise regularly than to exercise sporadically. So you will want to be truly ready before taking the plunge.

ESSENTIAL

It is perfectly fine if you need more than the standard six to eight weeks often quoted before regaining enough strength to exercise again. I would encourage you, however, to ask yourself if you are setting up emotional roadblocks to your recovery. Sometimes it's sheer timing. Just when you are physically ready to exercise—something in life happens.

Perhaps you are going back to work just as you are physically ready to exercise. You need to get this one more hurdle done before you leap into a fitness routine. Perhaps your older children are out on break as soon as your bleeding stops. You might need a bit more time, or until they head off to school again.

No matter what the timing, it is important that you take into consideration all of these factors. There is not one right answer. Once you have the physical go-ahead from your practitioners, the rest will fall into place. It cannot be rushed and does have a mind of its own. Just be sure to stay on top of it and not let it slip away without much thought.

Developing a Plan for Your New Body

Your postpartum plan is probably something you started thinking about before your pregnancy was through. While it is always great to have some vision of where you are going and where you want to be, you may find that the reality of being a new mom is more than you bargained for. Remember always to be flexible and keep everything in mind when trying to find your way.

Once you have the physical permission and the lifestyle adjustments necessary to exercise, it is time to figure out the practicality of it all—the how, what, where, when, and whys are what really matter. It is also important to realize that the answers to these questions may change as you adapt to your new life and new roles. You should also expect to adapt nearly everything you are doing, which is where that flexibility comes in handy.

How to Exercise?

You need to assess body problems that may be issues while exercising postpartum. This can include testing for diastasis recti, or separated abdominal muscles.

It is highly recommended that you check your recti muscles along the central seam, directly down the center of your abdominal muscle, for a separation, known as diastasis recti. This condition can occur for many reasons, pregnancy being one of them. However, you can work on this diastasis recti during pregnancy to help lessen its effects and decrease the width. (Please see Chapter 10 on how to check for diastasis recti.)

What you did prior to giving birth may be fine. You might start there with a reduced workout and slowly build it back up to where you were prior to giving birth. Then you can go forward and expand upon that base. Maybe you sense it is time for change. There are many programs designed for new mothers; in fact, there are probably more for new mothers than there are for expectant mothers.

Where to Exercise?

Where you exercise will depend on what exercises you choose. You might exercise at home in the living room while watching a taped class. Maybe you will walk around the neighborhood with some friends. Consider joining a walking club at a local mall or even a team that is taking people on to train for short runs like a 5K. You also have the option of going to a gym or other organized sporting arena.

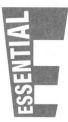

Learning to deal with change is never easy. Knowing what to expect from your body can help make this adjustment a bit easier. Realizing that you must have realistic expectations will be helpful in the road to recovery.

When to Exercise?

When to exercise is always a huge question. Try not to let your new little one add to that problem. Many new moms take classes with their babies, like the stroller aerobics or other classes. You might find that your husband is more than willing to watch junior for an hour when he comes home while you walk or do an aerobics class. If you've gone back to work, consider using your lunchtime for a quick trot around the block. Or even better maybe you could bike, jog, or walk to work. Always make time to exercise.

Why Exercise at All?

That question is one that only you have the answer for. You know the physical and emotional benefits. You can be told what they are all day long. In the end, it will come down to what really motivates you to exercise. That answer will be different for everyone. Ⓔ

Chapter 20

Finding Your Body after Birth

Giving birth is a life-altering experience. It also alters your body. The changes that came with pregnancy have receded, leaving you with a new form. Accepting your body and learning to work with it are key parts of the postpartum phase. Using exercise to help find the new you, and to alleviate stress and anxiety are perfect activities for new mothers.

Postpartum Weight Loss

One of the biggest things on your mind is probably losing the weight you gained while you were pregnant. Remember that it took your body nine months to gain the weight, which was distributed in a certain manner to help promote pregnancy and breastfeeding. Now, the process of losing the weight will also need to proceed in a particular fashion. You really need to focus on giving yourself the time to lose the weight, without pressure from your own ideas or from those around you.

Exercise and Diet Roles

Exercise will play a large component in your quest to lose the weight after your baby is born. However, you also need to focus on taking care of your body. This includes watching what you eat.

Also, your diet postpartum does not necessarily need to be one of self-sacrifice, but you do need to pay attention to healing your body and feeding your baby if you're breastfeeding. This doesn't mean you can't have sweets and high-fat foods. Just as with any other time in your life, you may want to eat foods that are not the best choices but in moderation.

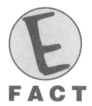

FACT

It takes about 500 to 1,000 calories a day to supply milk for your baby. If you are trying to lose weight, eating your normal diet will likely be sufficient for you to see a weight loss, because these calories are not typically included in your daily expenditure, as far as your body is concerned. However, any severe form of calorie restriction can cause a depletion in milk supply at any point in lactation. Weight loss attempts in the first six weeks are never recommended as that is when you are building the basis of your milk supply.

Exercise and Breastfeeding

Breastfeeding is a great start not only for your baby but for you as well. You are perfectly able to nurse and exercise. In fact, nursing moms are more likely to lose their pregnancy weight than those who do not nurse.

During pregnancy, part of the fat stores your body accumulates is in preparation for nursing. These fat stores are not called upon until after the baby is born and lactation begins. You may find, as some mothers do, that these stores are not tapped into right away. They are a protective mechanism by your body to protect your baby's food supply should you find yourself in a situation where you are starving. However, these fat stores are best removed by breastfeeding. The other alternative is liposuction!

During the first two months postpartum, you will find that weight loss tends to be dramatic. It is best for you to limit your weight loss while nursing to about 4 pounds a month after the initial postpartum period is over. This is to help protect your milk supply.

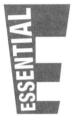

If you are breastfeeding, you may think you have to avoid eating certain foods or that you must eat certain foods. Neither of these statements is true. Breastfeeding moms can usually eat whatever they want to eat. Some babies may be sensitive to certain foods, however. Talk to your pediatrician if you think your baby is one of these babies.

Identifying Areas That Need Attention

During the initial days and weeks after birth, you might believe that everything needs your attention when it comes to your body. Remember, it took your body nine months to grow your baby and the changes were slow, not drastic. It really is best to approach postpartum changes in the same manner. The good news is that in many ways they are faster than the nine months. Once you are ready (mentally, physically, emotionally) to exercise, you can do more than you could during pregnancy because of fewer restrictions. You then control the amount of change to a degree that you could not during pregnancy. Patience is still a virtue in this arena.

The uterus is an amazing organ. It started out weighing about 3 ounces and being about the size of your fist before you were pregnant. As your baby grew, your uterus expanded and grew to help accommodate and nourish your baby. At term, your uterus weighed about 3 pounds and measured about 10 inches by 14 inches. That's quite a change! While it took nine months for the original change, the process of involution (your uterus returning to its prepregnancy size), usually takes about six weeks, no matter how you gave birth.

Your breasts also grew during pregnancy to accommodate the tissues needed for nursing your baby after birth. Choosing a good bra will help give you added support in this area. This is a must for a good postpartum workout.

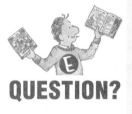

QUESTION?

Will exercise affect my breast milk?
There have been some reports that breast milk is higher in lactic acid after exercise. This does not affect your baby's ability to nurse, nor does it appear to cause the baby to have an aversion to post-exercise breast milk. There is no harm in nursing your baby immediately after exercising.

The skin on your abdomen might be another concern you have. Immediately after giving birth you feel really thin! Then you stand up and see the skin hanging there and moving too much like gelatin for your comfort. The skin will begin to shrink back and most women report that it does eventually get most of its tone back. Certain exercises can help speed this process up.

The angry red stretch marks will begin to fade as well. By six months, they are usually quite silvery and barely noticeable. Lotion will keep the skin lubricated, but there isn't a special potion out there to remove stretch marks.

Separation of the Abdominal Muscles

It is highly recommended that you check your rectus muscles along the central seam, directly down the center of your abdominal muscle, for a separation, known as a diastasis recti. This condition can occur for many reasons, pregnancy being one of them. However, you can work on this diastatsis recti during pregnancy to help lessen its effects and decrease the width.

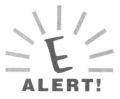

Postpartum support belts can be very beneficial. This is especially true if you're having trouble remembering to hold in your abdominal muscles as you work out or go about your day. If you gave birth to multiples or suffered a severe overdistention for a variety of reasons, it might be even more helpful.

When to Begin Your Postpartum Program

The last thing on your mind as your cradle your new baby is probably exercise, though every single movement you do, even in these first few hours, will help you on the road to your physical and mental recovery. And the sooner you get started, the better off you will be!

Doing certain breathing techniques can help you learn to fill your no-longer-impeded lungs. It can also help you avoid complications, like blood clots, particularly if you gave birth via cesarean surgery. Kegel exercises are awesome for initiating a return of blood flow to your perineum. This also can help decrease pain and swelling and promotes healing in this area.

Special Exercises for Cesarean Moms

Having a surgical birth can leave you physically exhausted and in pain. Good pain control the first few days after surgery will help you achieve a faster recovery. New cesarean moms often neglect adequate pain relief. They desire not to be medicated so they can enjoy their baby, and many are often concerned about the effect of medication on breast milk.

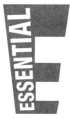

If you've had a cesarean birth, keep in mind that you are not only experiencing the normal postpartum occurrences, such as changes in hormones and bleeding, but you are also recovering from major abdominal surgery.

The First Few Days after Surgery

The exercises for the first few days after surgery really focus on prevention of complications. Learning to breathe after an abdominal incision is not as easy as it sounds. However, the more deep breathing you do, the less likely you are to have complications. As you hold your incision with your hands or brace it with a pillow, inhale. Put enough pressure or support on your abdomen so that you don't feel your incision will open. Do this frequently in the first few days to help prevent problems with your recovery.

In addition, try these exercises:

■ Walking

The first few times you get up to walk after surgery are likely to be slow and painful. Use a pillow or your hands to brace your incision. While it may feel like your organs are going to fall out, you have many layers of stitches inside your body, as well as external stitches or staples. It doesn't sound like a lot of fun, but getting up and walking will speed your recovery. The first day or two you will need someone to help you. By the second postpartum day you will probably be asked to walk around the postpartum floor or nurses station several times a day.

■ Abdominal Tightening

As you lie in bed, or on the floor, have your knees bent and your feet flat on the floor. Tighten your buttocks and press your lower back into the bed or floor. As you inhale, imagine pulling your stomach down through your back to the floor or bed. Hold for up to five seconds. You can repeat this up to ten times.

■ Leg Slides

Lie down on your back, and bend your right leg up, leaving your left leg flat on the bed, toes up. Slide your right leg down to rest next to your left leg. Slide it back up to the bent position again. Repeat this exercise five to ten times. Then repeat it with your left leg. If you're more comfortable, try holding a pillow over your incision while you do this exercise.

The Second Week after Surgery

As your recovery progresses you will be able to do more and more. Do keep in mind that you have had major abdominal surgery, in addition to the joys of postpartum and new motherhood. Be sure to ask for help around the house and remember to allow others to do what they can. The less you do now, the faster you will heal completely.

These more advanced exercises can be tried in the second week postpartum:

■ Pelvic Roll

Lie on your back with your feet together. Your knees should be bent. As you hold your knees together, bring them up toward your chest. Roll them to your right side. Slowly roll them to your left side. This is a gentle rocking motion. You should avoid any jerking or bouncing while doing this. If this exercise pulls on your incision, stop doing it immediately. Repeat this up to ten times on each side.

■ Abdominal Strengthening

Lie down on your back with your feet together and knees slightly bent. Crisscross your arms over your abdomen, grabbing your waist on the opposite side.

As you lift your head, pull your arms together, thus pulling your stomach muscles toward each other. Try to imagine that you have an apple under your chin to ensure proper head alignment during this exercise. Don't go too far up; your shoulders should barely leave the ground when doing this. Hold the pose for three to five seconds and then relax your head and arms to the original starting position. Repeat this exercise up to five times.

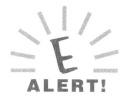

ALERT!

During the first two weeks' postpartum, you should refrain from walking the stairs more than about once a day. You should not drive your car. Do not lift anything heavier than your baby.

The Third Week after Surgery

By now you probably feel much better, though you still have some lingering pain and tension. Be sure to listen to your body and watch your incision. Add exercises slowly to the previous week's exercises as you build your body back up:

■ Pelvic Tilt

After about two weeks, you can begin to do your pelvic tilts. Assume an all-fours position, on your hands and knees. Think of holding your back in its natural alignment (see **FIGURE 5-7**, p. 61). Then tuck only your pelvis in, bringing your pubic bone toward your neck. Be sure to move only your pelvis (see **FIGURE 5-8**, p. 61). If it helps, have someone hold your pelvis so that you can learn to isolate this area. Later this exercise can be done in different positions. You need to do two sets of up to ten repetitions of the pelvic tilts. Later, you can add more to each set of repetitions.

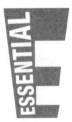

The area of your incision may feel numb. Some women report that this numbness lasts for years, if not permanently. You might also feel like there is itching below the skin. This is also normal. The surgery requires that muscles and therefore nerves be cut, thus causing this damage. Always ask your doctor or midwife if your incision is bothering you.

After the beginning exercises of breathing and abdominal tightening of the first few days, you will slowly begin to feel better. Your recovery will usually not be as fast as your vaginal birth counterparts, but you can affect the length of time you take to recover by not doing too much.

Once you've been given the go-ahead for exercising, you will want to pay particular attention to your abdominal muscles. Even beyond normal separation from pregnancy, your muscles have been surgically cut. If you had a low transverse or bikini incision, you will not have as severe of an abdominal problem than if you required a classical or vertical incision. This type of incision will damage more muscles.

Exercises to Regain Body Control

The best exercise for you and your postpartum body will be the one that you stick to on a regular basis. Identifying the problem areas will assist you in feeling more in control of your body.

Your new body will likely be very different from what you imagined. There will be some areas that are better than you anticipated, while others will be more problematic than you expected.

Many women judge their recovery based on the scale, but this is not the appropriate way to judge how well you are getting back into shape. Even after you've lost the weight you've gained in pregnancy, your body is likely to be different.

Instead, it's best to focus on how you're feeling and how you are looking. The more fit you are, the better you will feel, mentally as well as physically. You will have fewer sleep and digestive troubles. You will be able to feel good while exercising and actually miss it when you're unable to work out.

Sample Exercise Program

Here is a sample of some of the exercises that you can safely use during the postpartum period. There are more that you can do as well, but these should be familiar to you as they are from your pregnancy exercises. Slowly move them around and add new ones as you feel able to try them. Once approved for exercise, you can also start focusing on increasing your heart rate and you don't have to worry as much about overheating as you did while you were pregnant.

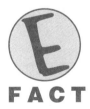

FACT

Areas like your hips and ribs will have expanded to accommodate your uterus as it grew. These areas will likely continue to be slightly larger than prior to pregnancy, no matter how hard you work.

Stretches

Try these stretches:

■ Neck Stretch

Stand with your feet shoulder-width apart. Let your shoulders be held up and back. The crown of your head should be pulling upward. Slowly let your chin drop to your chest and hold it there for five to ten seconds. Return your head to the neutral position. Slowly let your left ear rest on your left shoulder, again holding it for five to ten seconds. Repeat this with your right side. It is okay if you can't hold your head all the way down. Move until you feel the stretch, but without pain. Do this series three to five times.

■ Chest Stretch

Stand with your feet about shoulder-width apart, pelvis tucked in, and abdominals held tightly. Spread your arms to each side, at shoulder level (see **FIGURE 6-3**, p. 79). Slowly curl your back forward, while bringing your arms forward as well. Allow your head to go forward slowly with this motion but try to keep the tension from your neck (see **FIGURE 6-4**, p. 79). As you return to a standing pose, spread your arms back to your side and feel the stretch in your chest. To ensure you feel this stretch, pull your shoulder blades together behind your back. Repeat this ten times.

Birth Ball Exercises

■ Bridge on Ball

While sitting on a birth ball (see **FIGURE 6-7**, p. 83), slowly walk your feet in front of you until the ball is between your shoulder blades (see **FIGURE 6-8**, p. 83). Keep your ankles in line with your knees and be careful not to extend your knees farther than your toes. Keep your feet as wide apart as needed to maintain your balance. When you achieve this balance, squeeze your abdominal muscles, gluteal muscles, and hamstrings as you breathe and hold the position for three to five breaths. Lower your hips after you've achieved that number of breaths, then assume the position again. Repeat it ten times.

■ The Figure Eight

Sitting upright on your ball, place your hands on your hips. Imagine what a figure eight looks like. Begin your figure eight, leading with the left hip, going to the right, and backward diagonally, still with your left hip. Then switch to lead with your right hip, up and back until your figure eight is completed.

Wall Exercises

■ Wall Pushups

Facing the wall, place your hands palm down on the wall; walk your feet backward, away from the wall (see **FIGURE 5-1**, p. 58). Slowly bend your elbows, bringing your upper body closer to the wall (see **FIGURE 5-2**, p. 58). Do about ten repetitions of the exercise. Remember to keep your spine in the proper alignment while doing this exercise.

■ Posture Retraining

Place your back against the wall; slowly walk your feet forward until they are 6 to 8 inches in front of you. Press your glutes, shoulder blades, and the back of your head into the wall (see **FIGURE 5-3**, p. 59). Slowly raise your arms at a 90-degree angle, bent elbow to the wall, and press them to the wall as well. Slowly raise your arms, keeping them on the wall, above your head (see **FIGURE 5-4**, p. 59).

Standing Exercises

■ Knee Bends

Stand with your feet slightly greater than shoulder-width apart. Begin by tilting your pelvis and begin to bend your knees. Keep your head remaining upright and don't move your feet on the floor. Return to your original pose. This is a slow motion. Do not jerk or bounce. Repeat this exercise for a total of ten repetitions.

■ Knee Raises

Stand with your feet slightly greater than shoulder-width apart, placing your hands on your hips or at your sides (see **FIGURE 6-1**, p. 78). While maintaining your proper posture, lift your right knee until it is at about a 90-degree angle (see **FIGURE 6-2**, p. 78). Slowly lower your leg. Repeat this exercise for a total of ten repetitions and then switch knees for another ten repetitions. For a variety, alternate each leg for a total of ten repetitions each leg.

Sitting/Kneeling Exercises

■ Seated Row

Sitting on the floor with a flex band wrapped around your feet at the middle of the band, hold one end of the band in each hand (see **FIGURE 6-9**, p. 84). Your palms should be facing the floor. Pull the bands to your chest. Hold this for one count. Slowly release the tension in the band, returning to the original pose. Repeat this rowing motion ten times.

■ Cat Balance

While kneeling on the floor, pull in your abdominal muscles and breathe naturally. As you exhale extend your right leg and left arm. Think about extending each limb as far as you comfortably can. Hold this pose for three to five breaths. Repeat ten times on each side.

Lying Exercises

■ Hip Abduction Lying

Lie down on your back with your knees bent, feet flat on the floor, and your shoulders and hips firmly on the floor. Place your right ankle on your left knee. Bring your left knee toward your chest by grabbing your left thigh with your left hand (see **FIGURE 5-11**, p. 63). Hold this for about five seconds. Repeat on the opposite side.

■ Neck Roll-ups

Lie on the floor on your back as flat as you can. Tilt your pelvis up, so that your spine is flat on the floor. Slowly begin to curl your body up from the chin to the neck, bringing your head with your chin. Pull up until your shoulder blades are off the floor (see **FIGURE 5-10**, p. 62). Hold this pose for five to ten seconds. Repeat ten times.

Chapter 21

Exercising with Baby

Once your miracle arrives, your life is turned upside down. Rather than forget about spending time taking care of you, find a way to make your life work *with* Baby. This means finding the time to take care of your body in order to be strong, healthy, and mentally fit to take care of your new family.

Managing Exercise with Kids

We all have excuses as to why we can't exercise. Time is the biggest excuse found. We do not have time because of work. We do not have time because of other commitments. We do not have time because of family. The truth is we rarely make the time to exercise.

By making the time to exercise, we show others and ourselves our commitment to fitness. This will, in turn, influence your children as they grow up. As they see your commitment to exercise, they too will learn that it is an important part of life and that they must make time for themselves.

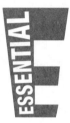

Besides exercise, breastfeeding is another way to help curb the problem of childhood obesity. While we know that breastfeeding has many benefits to you as a mother, there are also many benefits to your baby, many of which extend beyond those first few months. A reduction in obesity later in life is one of those benefits.

When to Exercise

Set aside some time each day to work out. This does not have to be an hour every day. It does not have to be at the same time, though that often helps when trying to establish a routine. Do not make the time you choose so late in the day that you are too exhausted, or that you allow other things to take precedence.

Sometimes you will want to exercise alone, without your new baby or other children. Perhaps the answer for this situation is to get up before your husband leaves for work to walk or do an exercise video. This often works well because it starts your day out on a positive note with one major thing already accomplished.

An alternative to this schedule would be to exercise when your husband comes home from work. The problem with waiting this late in the day is that we are usually tired at this point and less willing to get out and move. While the free time might be greatly appreciated, it takes a lot more motivation to get outside and move, rather than curl up and take a nap. If you choose this type of arrangement, be sure to find a way to stay motivated to get out and go.

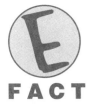

FACT

Even working out for twenty minutes four to five times a week is a great boost to your self-esteem and your fitness level. Remember that working out consistently is important. In fact, inconsistent exercise can be more hazardous than no exercise.

Another difficulty with late-in-the-day exercise is that your schedule may be interrupted by delays because of your husband's work schedule, the weather, or traffic. Try to find alternatives to do in case this happens. This always allows you the ability to do your exercise or workout, while still planning for contingencies.

Work Out with Your Baby

While the baby is still small, you might be able to work out with the baby present. Some moms use a swing or bouncy chair to entertain the baby while they throw in an aerobics or yoga tape. Your baby is usually entertained simply by watching you work out. You can talk to your baby while working out, a great way to check your exertion level! Babies enjoy the visual and auditory stimulation.

The use of a sling can also be beneficial while exercising. Using a sling or other infant carrier can allow you to get some forms of exercise done, while holding on to your little one. Try doing some light aerobics or stretching while carrying the baby this way. Try to keep one hand on the baby at all times to ensure his or her safety.

If you do not feel comfortable doing this, or prefer your workouts in solitary, naptime may be another time for you to try to squeeze in a workout. Not every baby will have a predictable naptime, so this may throw you off, but you can usually get in one workout every few days with most babies. You need to be prepared to get up and get moving as soon as the little one is down.

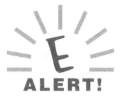

ALERT!

Be very careful while using your baby as a weight. If the baby resists or is fighting you in any way, immediately stop the workout. The workout should be a good experience for the baby as well as you. It also needs to be a safe experience.

Exercises Using Baby as a Weight

If you have a cooperative baby, you might be able to incorporate your baby into your workout. They can make great weights! This is often done when they are old enough to begin holding up their own heads, around two to three months of age, and it usually continues until they weigh too much to be lifted comfortably.

Sample Exercises with Baby

While there are many different things that you can make up on your own, there are a few that are often talked about. Here are some exercises to try with your baby:

■ Lying Biceps Curl with Baby

Lie on your back with your knees bent. Hold your baby under the arms, on your chest. The baby should be belly down. Lift your baby up toward the ceiling as you exhale. As you inhale, slowly lower your baby back to the starting position by lowering your elbows to your sides. Repeat this exercise for ten to twelve repetitions. A variation to this exercise is to move the baby up and over your head, then back down toward your knees, rather than simply a straight up-and-down motion. This will give a slight twist to the workout.

■ Biceps Curl with Baby

While sitting in a chair, place your baby facedown across your right forearm. Hold your baby across his chest with your left hand. Your right hand should hold the baby's left thigh or legs, near the buttocks (see **FIGURE 21-1**). Starting with your forearm parallel to the floor, lift the baby up toward your shoulder while holding the baby firmly with both hands (see **FIGURE 21-2**). You can do up to ten repetitions of this exercise. Switch the baby to your left forearm and begin the process again.

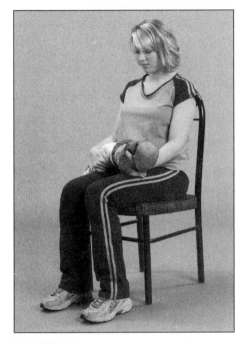

FIGURE 21-1
Biceps Curl with Baby—
Hang on tightly!

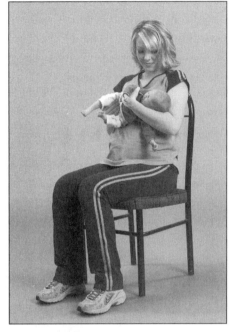

FIGURE 21-2
Seize the opportunity to gaze at
at your baby and interact

■ Leg Lifts with Baby

Sit on the floor or mat with baby lying down, facing you on your knees. Baby's chin should be between your knees. Hook your arms around Baby's back, and smile and talk to her. Slowly bring your feet off the floor, resting only on your buttocks. Be sure you feel stable enough to continue. Begin by raising your legs so that your legs are at a 45-degree angle from the knees. Repeat these leg lifts ten to twelve times. You can also switch and do single leg lifts with an older baby. Your baby needs to have some neck control to make this safe for her.

Enhance this exercise by playing with your baby. During your workout, feel free to sing and play games like peek-a-boo to keep Baby entertained. Keeping Baby happy will help you have more time to work out. This leads to a happier workout for all involved.

■ Squat

Now that you are used to doing squats, it's time to incorporate Baby! As you slowly lower your body, hold the baby in your arms, away from your body but facing you. Go down as far as you can, while keeping your heels on the floor. Do ten squats, holding each one five to ten seconds. Avoid bouncing in between or during squats. You can also incorporate your baby into other leg work, like lunges.

Finding Child Care While You Exercise

Sometimes the easiest solution to finding time to work out is finding adequate and appropriate child care. This can be done in a variety of ways. You might join a gym where child care is offered. You might work out a schedule with another mother to swap child care duties so that you can work out. You might even join or start a formal co-op to exchange child care.

Using the Buddy System

Not only can being a new mother be physically demanding, but also it can be isolating. Finding other new mothers out there who also desire exercise and yet lack time can be a great way to get your exercise and find some companionship. It can also be the answer to your workout woes.

If you know other mothers, that would be the place to start. Not only do you feel comfortable with these women, but also you probably will feel better leaving your baby in their care. They may even have a child of a similar age.

E ALERT!

Travel time can be a real problem with this plan. Finding someone close to home works best. Otherwise, you might be spending more time traveling around than working out. When this happens it leads to a decline in your motivation because of the effort it takes to make it happen.

The actual arrangements can vary from group to group. Perhaps you both gather at one house and take turns watching the babies while the other works out. Some moms choose to switch homes. Alternatively you can switch days. This gives one mom two days one week and three the next if you use a five-day a week schedule.

Starting an Exercise/Child Care Co-op

Perhaps you are feeling like a go-getter! If so, consider starting your own child care cooperative for the neighborhood, or among friends. This is a great way to get some time alone, and yet not worry about the expense. All you need to get going is three other moms. However, the more moms you have in your co-op the easier it can be.

The first step, after finding willing families, is to set up a meeting of all the moms (or dads). During this meeting, you need to agree upon the rules, the reimbursement, and other potential questions. Many co-ops use poker chips or paper money as currency, so you also need to decide how many to give each family at the start, how much time each will be worth, and so on. Discussing these issues up-front will help prevent problems in the future.

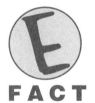

FACT

Having quarterly meetings and inviting new people to join your group are also good ways to grow your co-op and to keep misunderstanding to a minimum. Make sure members of each family are present at this meeting.

While this system can get complicated, it's also a great way to use the time for things other than exercise. The nice thing about doing it for exercise is that if your group is exercise-minded, you know you'll be returning the favor enough times to get in adequate amounts of exercise each week.

Special Programs for Moms and Babies

Sometimes there aren't many other options for a variety of reasons. Perhaps you do not know any other moms or do not trust the ones you do know. There are alternatives to using co-ops and friends to help you with child care while you exercise.

Some gyms have child care available on the premises. Check out these options when searching for the right gym. Ask questions about the facilities for children:

- At what age do you accept infants?
- Are the child care fees included in your membership payments?
- Do you need to schedule a time to work out or are you able to drop your child off?
- What is the sick child policy?
- Is there a time limit for your child?
- Is there a limit to the number of days or hours you can use each week?
- What is the student/child ratio?
- Are there multiple age groups in one class?
- Is there a space to nurse your baby?
- Are the workers trainer in CPR and other safety measures?
- Does the facility meet the basic state requirements to operate? (Look for certificate.)

Tour the child care facility to see if it feels warm and friendly to you. How do the staff workers relate to the kids? Try to talk to other parents who use the facility. This will give you an idea of how other parents feel about the care their child is getting and may serve to set your mind at ease.

One of the nice things about many on-site child care centers is that you are right there in the facility if you are needed for some reason. This may be the deciding factor in which workout facility you choose. It is also nice to have a facility that caters to the whole family and removes as many barriers as possible. You might even look ahead to see what they offer in the way of classes for younger children. Many gyms and fitness centers are expanding to include the entire family.

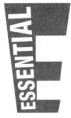

Jodi Levine of *daycare.about.com* recommends that a facility have no more than three infants per adult. The ratio for toddlers should be one adult for every five toddlers. Although the ratios will go up as the children become older, having other age groups mixed in with younger children does complicate matters.

Stroller Aerobics

There are also places that offer specific classes geared toward mother and baby. You might ask about Stroller Aerobics, a specialty class designed for postpartum mothers and babies of nearly any age.

Because the baby stays mostly in the stroller, you do not have to worry about how big your little one is getting. This is also great if you gave birth to more than one baby at a time, or if you have two babies who are close together in age. Simply put them all in the same stroller!

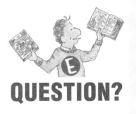

QUESTION?

Will I need a specific type of stroller?
Chances are the answer is no. Though some classes require strollers with brakes, there are usually very few requirements of your stroller. One of the fears many moms have is that they will need a fancy (and expensive) jogging stroller in order to be able to participate. Again, chances are good that your favorite everyday stroller will work just fine!

Many of these mother and baby stroller aerobics classes offer an aerobic portion, stretching, and even weight training. It's a great way to get out with other moms in your area, not to mention there is no concern about finding a baby-sitter or other child care arrangements.

Warm-up and Stretches

The majority of the classes begin with a warm-up and stretching exercises posed next to the stroller so that you can talk to or see your baby. You will do some neck stretches, and arm and leg stretches. You might do a warm-up like marching next to the stroller.

Once you've warmed up, you will do some fast-paced walking around the exercise area with the stroller, after a few laps you will start to add different steps. It might include knee lifts while walking, lunges, or other modifications to your stride such as taking wide steps (side ways).

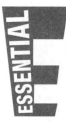

There are also many books and videos on the subject of mother and baby workouts. Each one will have a slightly different twist to it. Ask your friends and other new mothers if they have any recommendations. The key will be how well you and your baby like the program.

Repeaters

Interspersed within the exercises and strolling, you will do what our class calls *repeaters*. These are walking the length of the exercise area in a particular manner. Here is an example: eight steps, eight right-sided knee lifts, eight left-sided knee lifts; repeat this but add two sets of knee lifts; repeat but add three sets of knee lifts; repeat and take it down to two sets of knee lifts; return to the original set of one knee lift.

Turn the stroller around and head back in this manner: eight steps, eight jumping jacks, eight right-sided kicks, eight left-sided kicks; repeat five times or until you reach the end of your space.

Mat Workout

We end class with some mat work with weights. You work on your abdominal muscles, your arms, and then do some stretching and relaxation. Kids that are older can also be put to work helping to bring out the mats and smaller weights and helping put them away.

Many people are surprised at how strenuous the workout can be. It combines working your body while staying with your child. All in all, stroller aerobics is an awesome workout!

Mom and Baby Workout Classes

There are other mother and baby workout classes available. Yoga is usually a good option, as you can incorporate your baby into the poses. Some classes or instructors encourage you to do this. Find out if your yoga center or classes nearby offer specific mom and baby classes. If not, ask the instructor if he or she would mind if you brought your baby to class.

You can work with your instructor ahead of time to see what modifications are needed to assist you in making the class go smoothly. Usually the younger the baby, the better this plan works out. If you find the instructor is unable or unwilling to help you during class, ask if he or she would assist you after a class so that you can try to do this on your own.

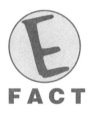

FACT

There are also programs that are designed with baby exercise only in mind. These classes can be great fun and most families report really enjoying them. The downfall for you is that you don't get the exercise you need from these classes.

Other Ways to Exercise with Your Baby

There are other ways to work out with your baby. These go beyond weight training. They are also often things you have done before.

Walking and Hiking

Walking and hiking are good exercises to do with Baby. The baby can stay in a sling or another type of infant carrier while you walk or hike. The added weight will provide you with more resistance and therefore a greater workout! When your baby is older, you can even do a backpack for your little one. They typically love being close to you and yet able to look around at their surroundings.

Water Aerobics

Water aerobics might be a good option for you and your little one. Try taking your baby to the pool and simply moving around. Remember, water provides more resistance and, therefore, even walking in water is a good workout. Moving your baby through the water, as you talk or play with him or her, provides some great interaction time as well.

Just remember finding time to work out is not always easy. There are many things you can do to find the time to work out. By taking care of yourself and your body you give your baby a healthy mother. This is a wonderful gift and one every child needs. Your baby will learn from you the value of working out and staying healthy. You are influencing the next generation to take care of their bodies as you are doing now. Ⓔ

Appendix A

Resources

Exercise-Related Organizations

American Council on Exercise (ACE)
4851 Paramount Drive
San Diego, California 92123
Phone: ✆ (858) 279-8227 or ✆ (800) 825-3636
Fax: ✆ (858) 279-8064
✐ *www.acefitness.org*

ACE has more than 45,000 active instructors currently working. They offer certification in the following areas: Personal Trainer, Group Fitness Instructor, Lifestyle & Weight Management Consultant, and Clinical Exercise Specialist. Look here for information on local trainers and facilities.

Aerobics and Fitness Association of America (AFAA)
15250 Ventura Boulevard, Suite 200
Sherman Oaks, CA 91403-3297
Phone: ✆ 1-888-968-7263
✐ *www.afaa.com/*
Contact: ✐ *ContactAFAA@afaa.com*

AFAA has certified more than 150,000 instructors since 1983. They offer continuing education and preparation for certification and information on locating instructors in your area as well as facilities.

American College of Sports Medicine (ACSM)
P.O. Box 1440
Indianapolis, IN 46206-1440
Phone: ✆ (317) 637-9200
✐ *www.acsm.org*

ACSM's goal is to integrate new science and information into the world of fitness.

Pregnancy-Related Organizations

Active Birth Centre
25 Bickerton Road, London N19 5JT
Tel: (44) 020 7281 6760
Fax: (44) 020 7263 8098
✐ *www.activebirthcentre.com*
Contact: ✐ *mail@activebirthcentre.com*

The Active Birth Centre promotes healthy views of pregnancy and birth. They encourage prenatal exercise and fitness and the use of active labor techniques.

American Academy of Husband Coached Childbirth (Bradley Method)
BOX 5224
Sherman Oaks, CA 91413-5224
Phone: 800-4-A-BIRTH
✐ *www.bradleybirth.com*

The Bradley Method of childbirth includes the use of deep relaxation and breathing with the help of the husband or partner through the labor process. The classes emphasize prenatal nutrition and exercise and their influence on a healthy pregnancy.

American College of Nurse Midwives (ACNM)
818 Connecticut Avenue, NW, Suite 900
Washington, D.C. 20006
Phone: ✆ (202) 728-9860
Fax: ✎ (202) 728-9897
✐ *www.midwife.org*

ACNM certifies nurse midwives (CNM) throughout the United States. They focus on the care of low-risk women through pregnancy and birth as well as other time periods of life. Well woman care is their specialty.

American College of Obstetricians and Gynecologists (ACOG)
409 12th Street, S.W.
P.O. Box 96920
Washington, D.C. 20090-6920
✐ *www.acog.org*

ACOG is the premiere organization for obstetricians and gynecologists. They manage the post–medical school training and certification of this specialty. These physicians are trained in the care of the woman during all stages of life.

Doulas of North America (DONA)
P.O. Box 626
Jasper, IN 47547
Phone: 888-788-DONA
✐ *www.dona.org*

DONA is the leading organization that certifies birth and postpartum doulas. A doula can assist the family before, during, or after birth. Using a doula has been shown to decrease the incidence of many complications of labor and postpartum, including cesarean section and postpartum depression.

International Cesarean Awareness Network (ICAN)
1304 Kingsdale Avenue
Redondo Beach, CA 90278
Phone: ✆ (310) 542-6400
✐ *www.ican-online.org*

ICAN works toward the prevention of unnecessary cesareans and the emotional and physical recovery from cesareans.

International Childbirth Education Association (ICEA)
P.O. Box 20048
Minneapolis, MN 55420
Phone: ✆ (952) 854-8660
✐ *www.icea.org*

ICEA trains childbirth educators as well as prenatal fitness instructors throughout the world. Their Web site offers a search to help you find local instructors.

Lamaze International
2025 M Street, Suite 800
Washington, D.C. 20036-3309
Phone: ✆ (202) 367-1128
✐ *www.lamaze-childbirth.com*

Lamaze International is the leading certifying organization for childbirth educators. Promoting normal birth is the core of their philosophy as they train educators worldwide. Their site offers a directory, articles, and other interactive features.

Books

Active Birth by Janet Balaskas, McGraw Hill, 1983

Balaskas is the founder of the Active Birth Centre in England and is also a birth activist there. Her book encourages women to use exercise and movement throughout pregnancy in order to prepare the body for the active work of giving birth.

Eat Well, Lose Weight While Breastfeeding by Eileen Behan, Villard Books, 1992

While breastfeeding does promote weight loss, the balance between keeping your baby well fed and losing weight can be a difficult one to maintain. Here's a different approach to the age-old question of how do you lose weight after pregnancy?

Essential Exercises for the Childbearing Year by Elizabeth Noble, New Life Images, 4th Edition, 2003

Ms. Noble is a physical therapist and the movement of the body is her specialty. She focuses on pregnancy fitness and how to stay healthy and fit while living a normal life during pregnancy. The book also includes information on proper body alignment and dealing with everyday questions like how to pick up older children and other posture questions.

Exercising Through Your Pregnancy by Dr. James Clapp III, Addicus Books, 1st Edition, 2002

Dr. Clapp is a leading researcher on pregnancy exercise and fitness. His work has won awards for the advances in maternal fitness. This book emphasizes the science behind the approval for exercising throughout pregnancy, including addressing tough issues like the serious athlete and exercise during pregnancy.

From Baby to Bikini by Greg Waggoner, Warner Books, 1999

A personal trainer shares his ideas on getting rid of the post-baby flab. From exercise to nutrition, Mr. Waggoner shares his personal philosophy of fitness after your baby arrives.

The Pilates Pregnancy by Mari Winsor, Perseus Publishing, 2001

This book is a very concise book of Pilates exercises for each trimester, including photos.

The Pregnancy Exercise Book by Judy Di Fiori, Harper Resource, Spiral Edition, 2000

This spiral-bound book is a great view of exercises for each trimester. The photos are clear and the text succinct. The binding makes it easy to prop up while you work out.

Web Sites

Childbirth.Org

✍ *www.childbirth.org*

This pregnancy Web site is dedicated to helping you maintain a healthy pregnancy. There are many informative articles on all aspects of pregnancy and fun programs including the boy or girl quiz and birth plan creator.

Exercise Guide at About

✍ *http://exercise.about.com*

Learn more about exercise for all walks of life, including pregnancy and postpartum.

Fit Pregnancy

✍ *www.fitpregnancy.com*

Fit Pregnancy is based on a magazine of the same name. Here you will find pregnancy fitness- and wellness-related articles.

Pregnancy Fitness Visitor Center

✍ *www.workoutsforwomen.com/pregnancy_ fitness_visitor_center.asp*

Here you'll find some basic workouts for pregnant women, with quick, easy descriptions and photos to help you along.

Pregnancy Guide at About

✍ *http://pregnancy.about.com*

Pregnancy-related articles including a pregnancy calendar, belly gallery, and other pregnancy fitness-related resources.

Running Guide at About

✍ *http://running.about.com*

This site contains information on the sport and art of running and jogging.

Swimming Guide at About

✍ *http://swimming.about.com*

Visit the swimming site at About.com for more information on swimming before, during, and after pregnancy.

Walking Guide at About

http://walking.about.com

Your walking guide for every avenue of life. Includes the 10-week Walk of Life program.

Appendix B

Sample Workouts for Pregnancy

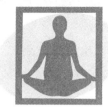

Each trimester of pregnancy has different workout needs. Here are some sample weeks for you to rotate during each trimester. There are a couple of different ways to use these weeks. You can simply rotate them in order, doing week one, followed by week two, then week three, and then start over. You can pick one week's schedule and do that repeatedly. You can decide each week which schedule to follow, or you can create your own. However, remember to always listen to your body when choosing your workout routine.

The First Trimester

Week One

Sunday:	Walk 20–60 minutes
Monday:	Aerobics 30–60 minutes
Tuesday:	Walk 20–60 minutes
Wednesday:	Rest
Thursday:	Aerobics 30–60 minutes
Friday:	Sport of your choice
Saturday:	Aerobics 30–60 minutes

Week Two

Sunday:	Yoga 30–60 minutes
Monday:	Aerobics 30–60 minutes
Tuesday:	Rest
Wednesday:	Yoga 30–60 minutes
Thursday:	Aerobics 30–60 minutes
Friday:	Rest
Saturday:	Aerobics 30–60 minutes

Week Three

Sunday:	Weight Training 30–45 minutes
Monday:	Aerobics 30–60 minutes
Tuesday:	Rest
Wednesday:	Aerobics 30–60 minutes
Thursday:	Swimming 45 minutes
Friday:	Rest
Saturday:	Aerobics 30–60 minutes

The Second Trimester

Week One

Sunday:	Yoga 45–60 minutes
Monday:	Aerobics 30–60 minutes
Tuesday:	Walk 20–60 minutes
Wednesday:	Rest
Thursday:	Aerobics 30–60 minutes
Friday:	Swimming 30–45 minutes
Saturday:	Aerobics 30–60 minutes

Week Two

Sunday:	Yoga 30–60 minutes
Monday:	Aerobics 30–60 minutes
Tuesday:	Rest
Wednesday:	Weight Training 30 minutes
Thursday:	Aerobics 30–60 minutes
Friday:	Rest
Saturday:	Aerobics 30–60 minutes

Week Three

Sunday:	Walk 20–45 minutes
Monday:	Aerobics 30–60 minutes
Tuesday:	Rest
Wednesday:	Aerobics 30–60 minutes
Thursday:	Yoga 30–60 minutes
Friday:	Rest
Saturday:	Aerobics 30-60 minutes

The Third Trimester

Week One

Sunday:	Yoga 30–45 minutes
Monday:	Aerobics 30–45 minutes
Tuesday:	Rest
Wednesday:	Walk 20–60 minutes
Thursday:	Aerobics 30–45 minutes
Friday:	Rest
Saturday:	Aerobics 30–45 minutes

Week Two

Sunday:	Yoga 30–45 minutes
Monday:	Aerobics 30–45 minutes
Tuesday:	Rest
Wednesday:	Yoga 30 minutes
Thursday:	Aerobics 30–45 minutes
Friday:	Rest
Saturday:	Aerobics 30–45 minutes

Week Three

Sunday:	Rest
Monday:	Aerobics 30–45 minutes
Tuesday:	Rest
Wednesday:	Aerobics 30–45 minutes
Thursday:	Yoga 20–30 minutes
Friday:	Rest
Saturday:	Aerobics 30–45 minutes

Index

THE EVERYTHING PREGNANCY ORGANIZER

By Marguerite Smolen

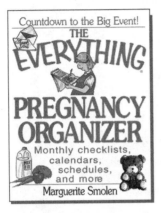

Countdown to the Big Event!
THE EVERYTHING PREGNANCY ORGANIZER

Monthly checklists, calendars, schedules, and more

Marguerite Smolen

Spiral bound paperback
$15.00 ($22.95 CAN)
1-58062-336-0, 336 pages

*T*he Everything® Pregnancy Organizer features everything a mother-to-be needs to get ready for a new baby. Complete with dozens of worksheets, checklists, pockets, and loads of helpful hints, this handy planner can help organize every aspect of your pregnancy. Arranged in an easy-to-use, month-by-month format, *The Everything® Pregnancy Organizer* is a calendar, journal, and medical resource. From keeping track of doctors' appointments and medical test results to creating shopping lists and choosing the perfect name, this organizer can become an expectant mom's best friend.

HISTORY

Everything® **American History Book**
Everything® **Civil War Book**
Everything® **Irish History & Heritage Book**
Everything® **Mafia Book**
Everything® **World War II Book**

HOBBIES & GAMES

Everything® **Bridge Book**
Everything® **Candlemaking Book**
Everything® **Casino Gambling Book**
Everything® **Chess Basics Book**
Everything® **Collectibles Book**
Everything® **Crossword and Puzzle Book**
Everything® **Digital Photography Book**
Everything® **Family Tree Book**
Everything® **Games Book**
Everything® **Knitting Book**
Everything® **Magic Book**
Everything® **Motorcycle Book**
Everything® **Online Genealogy Book**
Everything® **Photography Book**
Everything® **Pool & Billiards Book**
Everything® **Quilting Book**
Everything® **Scrapbooking Book**
Everything® **Soapmaking Book**

HOME IMPROVEMENT

Everything® **Feng Shui Book**
Everything® **Gardening Book**
Everything® **Home Decorating Book**
Everything® **Landscaping Book**
Everything® **Lawn Care Book**
Everything® **Organize Your Home Book**

KIDS' STORY BOOKS

Everything® **Bedtime Story Book**
Everything® **Bible Stories Book**
Everything® **Fairy Tales Book**
Everything® **Mother Goose Book**

EVERYTHING® *KIDS' BOOKS*

All titles are $6.95
Everything® **Kids' Baseball Book, 2nd Ed.** ($10.95 CAN)
Everything® **Kids' Bugs Book** ($10.95 CAN)
Everything® **Kids' Christmas Puzzle & Activity Book** ($10.95 CAN)
Everything® **Kids' Cookbook** ($10.95 CAN)
Everything® **Kids' Halloween Puzzle & Activity Book** ($10.95 CAN)
Everything® **Kids' Joke Book** ($10.95 CAN)
Everything® **Kids' Math Puzzles Book** ($10.95 CAN)
Everything® **Kids' Mazes Book** ($10.95 CAN)
Everything® **Kids' Money Book** ($11.95 CAN)
Everything® **Kids' Monsters Book** ($10.95 CAN)
Everything® **Kids' Nature Book** ($11.95 CAN)
Everything® **Kids' Puzzle Book** ($10.95 CAN)
Everything® **Kids' Science Experiments Book** ($10.95 CAN)
Everything® **Kids' Soccer Book** ($10.95 CAN)
Everything® **Kids' Travel Activity Book** ($10.95 CAN)

LANGUAGE

Everything® **Learning French Book**
Everything® **Learning German Book**
Everything® **Learning Italian Book**
Everything® **Learning Latin Book**
Everything® **Learning Spanish Book**
Everything® **Sign Language Book**

MUSIC

Everything® **Drums Book (with CD)**, $19.95 ($31.95 CAN)
Everything® **Guitar Book**
Everything® **Playing Piano and Keyboards Book**

Everything® **Rock & Blues Guitar Book (with CD)**, $19.95 ($31.95 CAN)
Everything® **Songwriting Book**

NEW AGE

Everything® **Astrology Book**
Everything® **Divining the Future Book**
Everything® **Dreams Book**
Everything® **Ghost Book**
Everything® **Meditation Book**
Everything® **Numerology Book**
Everything® **Palmistry Book**
Everything® **Psychic Book**
Everything® **Spells & Charms Book**
Everything® **Tarot Book**
Everything® **Wicca and Witchcraft Book**

PARENTING

Everything® **Baby Names Book**
Everything® **Baby Shower Book**
Everything® **Baby's First Food Book**
Everything® **Baby's First Year Book**
Everything® **Breastfeeding Book**
Everything® **Father-to-Be Book**
Everything® **Get Ready for Baby Book**
Everything® **Homeschooling Book**
Everything® **Parent's Guide to Positive Discipline**
Everything® **Potty Training Book**, $9.95 ($15.95 CAN)
Everything® **Pregnancy Book, 2nd Ed.**
Everything® **Pregnancy Fitness Book**
Everything® **Pregnancy Organizer**, $15.00 ($22.95 CAN)
Everything® **Toddler Book**
Everything® **Tween Book**

PERSONAL FINANCE

Everything® **Budgeting Book**
Everything® **Get Out of Debt Book**
Everything® **Get Rich Book**
Everything® **Homebuying Book, 2nd Ed.**
Everything® **Homeselling Book**

All Everything® books are priced at $12.95 or $14.95, unless otherwise stated. Prices subject to change without notice.
Canadian prices range from $11.95–$31.95, and are subject to change without notice.

Everything® **Investing Book**
Everything® **Money Book**
Everything® **Mutual Funds Book**
Everything® **Online Investing Book**
Everything® **Personal Finance Book**
Everything® **Personal Finance in Your 20s & 30s Book**
Everything® **Wills & Estate Planning Book**

PETS

Everything® **Cat Book**
Everything® **Dog Book**
Everything® **Dog Training and Tricks Book**
Everything® **Horse Book**
Everything® **Puppy Book**
Everything® **Tropical Fish Book**

REFERENCE

Everything® **Astronomy Book**
Everything® **Car Care Book**
Everything® **Christmas Book, $15.00 ($21.95 CAN)**
Everything® **Classical Mythology Book**
Everything® **Einstein Book**
Everything® **Etiquette Book**
Everything® **Great Thinkers Book**
Everything® **Philosophy Book**
Everything® **Shakespeare Book**
Everything® **Tall Tales, Legends, & Other Outrageous Lies Book**
Everything® **Toasts Book**
Everything® **Trivia Book**
Everything® **Weather Book**

RELIGION

Everything® **Angels Book**
Everything® **Buddhism Book**
Everything® **Catholicism Book**
Everything® **Jewish History & Heritage Book**
Everything® **Judaism Book**

Everything® **Prayer Book**
Everything® **Saints Book**
Everything® **Understanding Islam Book**
Everything® **World's Religions Book**
Everything® **Zen Book**

SCHOOL & CAREERS

Everything® **After College Book**
Everything® **College Survival Book**
Everything® **Cover Letter Book**
Everything® **Get-a-Job Book**
Everything® **Hot Careers Book**
Everything® **Job Interview Book**
Everything® **Online Job Search Book**
Everything® **Resume Book, 2nd Ed.**
Everything® **Study Book**

SELF-HELP

Everything® **Dating Book**
Everything® **Divorce Book**
Everything® **Great Marriage Book**
Everything® **Great Sex Book**
Everything® **Romance Book**
Everything® **Self-Esteem Book**
Everything® **Success Book**

SPORTS & FITNESS

Everything® **Bicycle Book**
Everything® **Body Shaping Book**
Everything® **Fishing Book**
Everything® **Fly-Fishing Book**
Everything® **Golf Book**
Everything® **Golf Instruction Book**
Everything® **Pilates Book**
Everything® **Running Book**
Everything® **Sailing Book, 2nd Ed.**
Everything® **T'ai Chi and QiGong Book**
Everything® **Total Fitness Book**
Everything® **Weight Training Book**
Everything® **Yoga Book**

TRAVEL

Everything® **Guide to Las Vegas**

Everything® **Guide to New England**
Everything® **Guide to New York City**
Everything® **Guide to Washington D.C.**
Everything® **Travel Guide to The Disneyland Resort®, California Adventure®, Universal Studios®, and the Anaheim Area**
Everything® **Travel Guide to the Walt Disney World Resort®, Universal Studios®, and Greater Orlando, 3rd Ed.**

WEDDINGS

Everything® **Bachelorette Party Book**
Everything® **Bridesmaid Book**
Everything® **Creative Wedding Ideas Book**
Everything® **Jewish Wedding Book**
Everything® **Wedding Book, 2nd Ed.**
Everything® **Wedding Checklist, $7.95 ($11.95 CAN)**
Everything® **Wedding Etiquette Book, $7.95 ($11.95 CAN)**
Everything® **Wedding Organizer, $15.00 ($22.95 CAN)**
Everything® **Wedding Shower Book, $7.95 ($12.95 CAN)**
Everything® **Wedding Vows Book, $7.95 ($11.95 CAN)**
Everything® **Weddings on a Budget Book, $9.95 ($15.95 CAN)**

WRITING

Everything® **Creative Writing Book**
Everything® **Get Published Book**
Everything® **Grammar and Style Book**
Everything® **Grant Writing Book**
Everything® **Guide to Writing Children's Books**
Everything® **Screenwriting Book**
Everything® **Writing Well Book**

Available wherever books are sold!
To order, call 800-872-5627, or visit us at everything.com

Everything® and everything.com® are registered trademarks of F+W Publications.